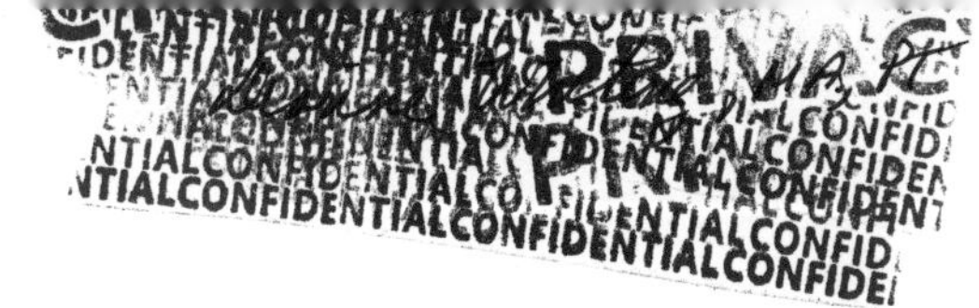

Fibromyalgia Syndrome

Physical Therapy Management

Kathryn Stogner Henderson, PT

Some of the illustrations in this guide were completed under contract by Scott Gee

Therapy Skill Builders®
a division of
The Psychological Corporation

555 Academic Court
San Antonio, Texas 78204-2498
1-800-228-0752

About the Author

Kathryn Stogner Henderson received her undergraduate degree from Duke University in Durham, North Carolina. After earning her degree, she joined the U.S. Army and received her certificate in physical therapy from the Medical Field Service School at Fort Sam Houston, Texas. She served another three years in the Army Medical Specialists Corps as a physical therapist and attained the rank of captain. Since leaving the army, Ms. Henderson has had a variety of clinical experiences, including flying into rural areas in eastern Colorado to provide therapy services, teaching prenatal and postpartum exercise classes, teaching childbirth preparation classes, and coordinating continuing education for a rehabilitation hospital. She has also worked as a staff therapist in home health, acute care, and rehabilitation hospital settings. In 1985, Ms. Henderson joined the physical therapy staff at SportsMed and Orthopaedic Rehabilitation in Carol Stream, Illinois. She took on additional responsibilities in 1992 as a consultant on disability assessment for MedEval Corporation in Lombard, Illinois. In 1994, she began work on the Master of Health Science in Physical Therapy degree through the University of Indianapolis.

Throughout her career, Ms. Henderson has been intrigued by myofascial pain and other soft tissue disorders. This interest led her to attend the first national seminar on Fibrositis/Fibromyalgia in Columbus, Ohio, in April 1990. In June of that year, Ms. Henderson helped establish a fibromyalgia support group in DuPage County, Illinois, and co-chaired the group for several years. She remains the primary contact person. In her clinical practice, she continues to try to find the best treatment program for her clients who suffer from fibromyalgia. Ms. Henderson lives in Wheaton, Illinois, with her family.

Contents

Introduction

As a physical therapist who graduated nearly 30 years ago, I often wonder how many people I have treated or consulted who had fibromyalgia before anyone was ever diagnosed with the fibromyalgia syndrome (FS). I shudder at the realization that there were many clients who tried to make us understand their plight yet we did not understand it. In fact, we probably treated them for whatever diagnosis they had been assigned and then puzzled over their poor outcomes. I do not recall specific clients, but I do recall hearing some tell me that they hurt all over (odd!), that the pain moved from one region of the body to another (unheard of!), that they were always tired (impossible!), or that they knew their problems all started with a motor vehicle accident (suspicious!).

Eventually, I became frustrated that pain, which appeared to be muscular in origin, could elude our therapy when we, as physical therapists, are so well educated about the musculoskeletal system. I started listening harder and trying to make the pieces fit into the structure I had been taught. I asked more experienced therapists about those tender "knots" in people's muscles. Occasionally they would have a helpful suggestion, the best of which was the advice to consult Dr. Travell's work. I felt that I had found the proverbial pot of gold because that first volume of Travell and Simon's *Myofascial Pain and Dysfunction* was such a treasure to me. But I still did not understand FS as a systemic condition and mistakenly considered the tender/trigger points and taut bands in the muscles to be the only characteristics of FS. Even so, many patients found good relief from the ischemic compression technique that Drs. Travell and Simon describe in their books. Therefore, their soft tissue compression technique became the cornerstone of my treatment approach for clients with FS.

My desire to understand the underlying mechanisms led me to other resources, such as research articles, a physiatrist who has FS, seminars, and newsletters. Through all of the searching, the most valuable resource has been, and continues to be, people who have FS, whether they are my clients, participants at support group meetings, or people who call on the phone seeking support of one kind or another. Their many stories have revealed to me certain commonalities in their symptomatology and patterns that are valid and unifying, despite the fact that there is not yet a diagnostic laboratory test.

In the past decade, many more of the characteristics have been elucidated. They include widespread muscular pain, tender/trigger points in the muscles, referred pain and paresthesia that do not confine themselves to dermatomal patterns, subjective swelling, irritable bowel and bladder, sleep disorders, fatigue, cognitive impairments, and general hypersensitivity to stimuli. The syndrome has been defined but the etiology remains mysterious. The onset is associated with several different triggering events, although, in some cases, it is insidious. Treatment also remains somewhat of a mystery, although we have made a lot of headway in helping clients find relief. Still, we do not know how to cure FS so it becomes a chronic issue, complete with the coping problems and vulnerability to depression that accompany any chronic medical problem.

In view of the fact that there are no definitive explanations of the etiology and course of FS, nor any decisive treatment protocol, you might question why someone would write a manual about FS. I think the very fact that there is so much confusion, skepticism, and misunderstanding about FS provides the reason for writing such a manual. Therapists who are faced with the challenge of assisting clients with FS need to have access to existing information, even though it is inconclusive. Therapists who read the most recent research and then use their ability to integrate this information with what they already know about the human body and the field of physical therapy, can provide better services to their clients and find greater satisfaction and less frustration in treating people with this diagnosis. Hopefully, this manual will save therapists valuable time by using the "wheel" that others have already developed. Beyond that step, I hope that therapists will use the valuable time they saved for listening to their clients more and for improving treatment methods. What does this manual offer to you as a physical therapist? The information on the history of the diagnosis, the various accepted definitions, the tender/trigger point phenomenon, and associated conditions will help you gain perspective on this mysterious syndrome. The section on research findings is fourfold in purpose:

- to expand your background knowledge
- to give you references for further study
- to provide you with some bases for treatment
- to demonstrate some of the significant distinctions
  between clients with FS and healthy individuals

I do not pretend that all the pertinent research is covered in these pages. There is a lot more information available for you to find. Nor do I assume that I have interpreted the research perfectly. My primary purpose is to present, not to interpret. I encourage you to interpret the findings based on your accumulated knowledge and experience. Then use all you have learned in the most important activity: treating your clients with FS.

I have devoted most of the manual to outlining the protocol that I have developed over the years. I am sharing this with you because I have had generally positive results. By no means do I believe that you must abide by this protocol to the letter. Human beings are too variable for that, not to mention the variability of the fibromyalgia syndrome. I alter this protocol to individualize it for each client. What I have attempted to do in the protocol section is to include the tools that I have found to be most beneficial. I am sure I have not included some that you may favor, in which case I would appreciate hearing from you about them. (You can send your ideas to me at 26 W 110 Durfee, Wheaton, IL 60187.) I cannot emphasize enough that I realize you already know a great deal about the human body and the effect of various types of exercises and modalities. My goal is to encourage you and assist you in using all of your knowledge and experience for treating this special client population who have some unusual treatment needs.

The people who have motivated me to write this book are the clients with FS. At least 2% of the general population, which is millions of people, suffer from FS. Many of these people have spent years searching for answers, undergoing surgeries, and trying alternative medicine when traditional medicine did not help. They have spent large sums of money and visited numerous medical professionals and, as a result, have become the subject of jokes about hypochondriacs. Not only have they lost credibility with their friends and families, but many have begun to doubt themselves as well. Some give in to despair, but many exhibit amazing strength of spirit and continue to push for answers and relief. They continue to hope, yet they still face struggles. They struggle with some medical professionals who know very little about FS and others who just do not care. They struggle with the reality that there is no cure. These good people have inspired me to do whatever I can to help them.

People with FS have more hope than ever before because increasing amounts of attention and money are being dedicated to the fibromyalgia syndrome. While we await a clear solution to the mystery of FS, we must do the best we can with the information we have. So, in the hope that therapists will be better enabled to assist clients with FS because of what they learn from this manual, the effort has been made. I acknowledge that the information available is incomplete and I hope that a revision of this manual will soon be needed because of significant new research findings. In fact, I would not be surprised if the name of the syndrome were changed one day to reflect the exact etiology when it has finally been found.

History of the Fibromyalgia Syndrome Diagnosis

It is helpful to know something about the evolution of the diagnosis of FS as we try to understand why we are seeing a greater consistency and frequency in the application of the FS diagnosis. This short summary of research findings demonstrates that more has been known about fibromyalgia for a longer period of time than many of us thought. Unfortunately, much of this information was ignored or simply not integrated for a long time.

FS is considered by some people to be a new disease or a "yuppie" disease caused by the stress of our times. It may surprise many readers to learn that aspects of FS have been described since the 17th century (Reynolds 1983). In 1843, Froriep used the term *muskelschwiele* (translated as muscle calluses) to describe palpable tender spots in muscles that were associated with pain (Travell and Simons 1983).

In 1904, Sir William Gowers published a paper in England on lumbago and coined the term *fibrositis* (Gowers 1904). In 1909, Osler, writing about muscular rheumatism, said that "It is by no means certain that the muscular tissues are the seat of the disease. It is a neuralgia of the sensory nerves of the muscles" (Smythe 1986). Gowers's term *fibrositis* replaced the term *muscular rheumatism*. It took the writings of Llewellyn and Jones to entrench Gowers's new term in medical terminology with the publication in 1915 of their book *Fibrositis*. According to Travell and Simons (1983), this book unfortunately served to confuse the meaning of the term.

In the 1930s, Lewis and Kellgren distinguished between skin pain and deep pain. They considered referred pain as stemming from deep structures and they included deep tenderness in this definition of referred pain. They also established that the referred pain usually traveled distally, sometimes quite a distance (Smythe 1986).

As long ago as the 1940s, researchers were publishing papers which indicated that a "central nervous system reflex disturbance" caused referred pain or that "there was a feedback mechanism between the trigger point and the central nervous system" (Travell and Simons 1983). In 1944, a researcher named Michael Kelly said, "Much that was obscure in fibrositis has been illuminated in the last six years, and one can hopefully expect that further studies, based upon the same scientific foundation, will give greater reality to that which still remains obscure" (Reilly and Littlejohn 1993a). However, the first controlled study of FS was not published until 1981 (Yunus et al. 1981).

Since the 17th century, at least 45 terms have been applied to this condition. In retrospect, it is obvious that semantics served to obscure the fact that many people were suffering from the same condition. This obscurity had a number of effects. One result of this lack of coordination of information was to rob patients of the support they could have provided each other. Another effect was that research was retarded or even neglected because it was thought that only a few people suffered with each of the "different" conditions. When it was realized that, in actuality, a lot of people were afflicted with this mysterious condition, then the interest in and urgency for research began. Listed below are some of the terms that have been used to diagnose patients with FS. Despite the fact that fibromyalgia syndrome (FS) is the currently accepted terminology, you will likely continue to see some of these terms used.

abdominal fibrositis	myalgic spots
affective spectrum disorder	myitis chronica
brachial fibrositis	myodysneuria
chest wall syndrome	myofascial trigger points
chronic rheumatism	myofasciitis
fibromyositis	myofibritis
fibropathic syndrome	myogelosis
fibrositic spots	myositis
fibrositis	nerve point
hypersensitive areas	nodular fibromyositis
idiopathic myalgia	nonarticular rheumatism
intercostal fibrositis	pain amplification syndrome
interstitial myofibrositis	panniculosis
invalidism	pressure points
lumbar fibrositis	psychogenic rheumatism
muscle hardenings	rheumatic myalgia
muscle indurations	rheumatic myositis
muscular fibrositis	scapulocostal syndrome
muscular rheumatism	tension rheumatism
muscular sciatica	traumatic myalgia
musculofascial pain	trigger points
myalgia	Valleix points

From the multitude of terms used to describe this syndrome, it is evident that no distinction was drawn between regional myofascial dysfunction and FS. Now that FS has been defined as a condition of widespread pain with bilateral presence of tender/trigger points as well as systemic problems, the distinction can be made more easily. "At this time, no specific cause of either fibromyalgia or myofascial trigger points has been established. However, clinically, myofascial pain caused by trigger points is primarily a focal dysfunction of muscle, whereas fibromyalgia is a systemic disease that also affects muscle" (Travell and Simons 1992). Travell and Simons (1992) also note that men and women are affected nearly equally by myofascial trigger points, whereas women with FS far outnumber men. They also point out that chronic myofascial dysfunction may be difficult to distinguish from FS.

Another problem in semantics occurs when some experts discriminate between primary fibromyalgia and secondary fibromyalgia. This labeling separates the cases in which symptoms seem to arise unprovoked (primary) and those cases in which symptoms begin to occur following trauma, a febrile illness, or surgery (secondary). Other experts do not distinguish between cases of FS in this manner.

Defining Fibromyalgia Syndrome

In order to treat a person with a medical condition and to help that person cope, it is necessary to have a full understanding of how the condition manifests in the body, what associated problems might arise, what the demographics are, and what stimuli affect the intensity and longevity of the symptoms. In other words, we need a definition. Finding an adequate definition for FS is not a simple task because the symptoms are widespread and variable and seem to be triggered by a number of different events. There is no confirming diagnostic lab test and there is no final consensus regarding a definition or diagnosis that can be drawn directly from research.

An attempt to standardize the definition and diagnostic criteria was made in 1990 by the American College of Rheumatology (ACR) (Wolfe et al. 1990). Included in their definition are the complaints found in 50% or more of the patients with FS they studied. These symptoms are:

- fatigue
- generalized pain
- sleep disturbance
- muscle stiffness
- headaches
- paresthesias

Other symptoms that were reported by individuals with FS include:

- muscle weakness
- cognitive impairment
- subjective swelling
- bladder irritability
- global anxiety
- dysmenorrhea
- local twitch response
- dermatographia
- hypersensitivity to environmental factors

Several other syndromes closely associated with FS are chronic fatigue syndrome, irritable bowel syndrome, mitral valve prolapse syndrome, sicca syndrome, and Raynaud's phenomenon.

Dr. George Waylonis, speaking at the 1992 National Seminar on Fibrositis/
Fibromyalgia in Columbus, Ohio, added a few other associated problems:

- plantar fasciitis
- chondromalacia
- bursitis
- vertigo
- sinus problems
- temporomandibular pain
- balance problems
- heat intolerance
- coccygeal pain
- burning feet
- concentration and memory problems
- premenstrual syndrome
- costochondritis
- fluid retention
- thyroid dysfunction

Since 1992, continuing research has expanded the view of FS. For example, a few
years ago cognitive impairment, global anxiety, and vulvodynia were not included
in anyone's description of FS, but they have been added by several experts recently.

Many people with FS relate that changes in their pain level often seem to correspond
to weather changes, physical activity, and stress. However, more often than not,
they seem to be at a loss to explain the variations in their pain level from day to
day or within a day's time.

While the combination of these clinical symptoms forms the basis for the definition
of FS, there seems to be general agreement that widespread pain and tender points
are the diagnostic criteria. According to the 1990 ACR Criteria for Classification
of FS, there must be a three-month history of widespread pain and there must be
pain in response to light pressure (4 kg) in 11 of 18 tender point sites in order for
the diagnosis of FS to be assigned (Wolfe et al. 1990). The ACR further defines
widespread pain to include all of the following: pain in the right and left sides of
the body, pain above and below the waist, and axial skeleton pain. The second
criterion for diagnosis deals with the tender points that are painful when about 4 kg
of pressure are applied. The person must describe this pressure as painful. If the
person describes this sensation as merely tender, it is not considered to be a positive
test. The 18 sites that are assessed include:

1. **occiput:** bilateral at the suboccipital muscle attachments

2. **low cervical:** bilateral, at the anterior aspects of the intertransverse spaces at
   C5-C7

3. **trapezius:** bilateral, at the midpoint of the upper borders

4. **supraspinatus:** bilateral, at the attachments above the scapular spine near the
   medial border

5. **second rib:** bilateral, at the second costochondral junctions, just lateral to the
   junctions on the upper surfaces

6. **lateral epicondyles:** bilateral, 2 cm distal to the epicondyles

7. **gluteal:** bilateral, in upper outer quadrants of buttocks in anterior fold of muscle

8. **greater trochanter:** bilateral, posterior to the trochanteric prominence

9. **knees:** bilateral, at the medial fat pad proximal to the joint line

This classification has been helpful in the determination of the FS diagnosis, but many clinicians feel that it is too rigid for clinical use. For instance, if an individual has only nine painful sites, should FS necessarily be excluded from the diagnosis? Would this person receive any treatment? On the other hand, the classification is critical in establishing valid and consistent participants in research studies. Such a standardized system of classification must be used in research so that the results of research are scientifically acceptable.

It should also be noted that with each of the tender sites, the diagnostician is instructed to assess both sides of the body. The word *bilateral* appears with each site. FS is a symmetrical condition even though the individual with FS may not realize it. Prior to the evaluation, the client might complain of pain on only one side of the body. During the evaluation, the person will become aware of the tender points on the contralateral side. Although the client is usually not happy to learn of these quiet or latent tender points, it is important to determine whether they exist and then to treat them. The fact that this condition is symmetrical has further implications if we accept Dr. I. Jon Russell's statement that "Generally in musculo-skeletal medicine, symmetry is considered to be an indication of a systemic process" (Russell 1994d, 76).

Another important aspect to note is that people with FS do not experience pain in response to pressure at control points, although these points may be tender (Campbell et al. 1983). Even though many individuals with FS describe themselves as hurting all over, there are definite, predictable tender point sites and definite control point sites. Control point sites are those that are not tender in people who are healthy or in people who have FS. Examples of control points are the belly of the deltoid, the volar aspect of the forearm, and the forehead (Bennett, Smythe, and Wolfe 1992). It is also important to recognize that people who are healthy do not experience pain when pressure is applied to the tender point sites that have been defined by the ACR.

Researchers often use a dolorimeter or algometer for tender point site assessment. Fischer (1987) studied 50 people who had no pain complaints using a pressure threshold meter (dolorimeter) with a 1 centimeter-squared surface and established average tolerances in a number of muscles. He generalized that intolerance to 3 kg of pressure or less indicates abnormality (Fischer 1987). This finding does not support the current use of 4 kg as the standard. Possibly the size of the head of the measuring instrument might have varied from instruments used by other researchers. A recent study demonstrated that changing the size of the head of the measuring instrument and changing the rate at which pressure was applied did, indeed, have an effect on a person's response to the pressure (White, McCain, and Tunks 1993).

Therefore, these researchers suggest that further studies on FS be done with the dolorimeter and that the head size and rate of application be standardized. Another variable might have been the degree of discomfort the subject felt before signaling intolerance.

Clinically, the use of the dolorimeter seems to be unnecessary as the therapist's palpatory skills and a helpful hint from I. Jon Russell, M.D., are sufficient. "Four kilograms of pressure is about what it takes to blanch the blood from the tip of the examiner's thumbnail when the palmar surface of the thumb is pressed firmly against an immovable object" (Russell 1994d). Dr. Russell and colleagues (1986) suggest the use of the following severity scale with the application of 4 kilograms of pressure:

- If there is no tenderness at a site, a "0" is given.
- If there is tenderness but no physical response, a "1" is given.
- If there is tenderness and some physical response, such as wincing or moving away, a "2" is given.
- If there is a "jump sign" or the patient sharply withdraws, a "3" is given.
- If the patient cannot allow the examiner to apply touch, a "4" is given.

A tender point index is obtained by adding up the scores for all 18 sites. This index can be ascertained again at a later time to assess the patient's progress or decline.

The intertester reliability of tender point determination has been investigated by blind studies. The degree of reliability is significant and valid for clinical use. The results showed a coefficient of 0.85 for reliability of the tender point threshold between two testers (Tunks et al. 1988). A confirming study was reported by Cott and colleagues (1992). Besides confirming the intertester reliability that Tunks and colleagues had found, Cott and colleagues also demonstrated that interrater reliability was the same for hand palpation as for dolorimetry. There was some discrepancy, however, between the two methods for defining points as tender. Cott and colleagues advised testers to use one method or the other in specific cases until further study has explained this discrepancy.

Another comment about the diagnosis of FS comes from Bernard Rubin (1994), who says, "The clinical characteristics of FS include widespread musculoskeletal aching, specific tender points, and a feeling of awakening unrefreshed in the morning. This common disorder has often been dismissed as imaginary or as a psychiatric form of malingering. Recent clinical, epidemiological, and basic science research has shown that fibromyalgia can be diagnosed with a careful history, appropriate laboratory tests, and the identification of specific tender points on physical examination." (His inclusion of laboratory tests is for the purpose of ruling out other disease processes. There is no diagnostic laboratory test for FS available yet.) Dr. Rubin (1994, 64) sums up the situation by saying that "Fibromyalgia is a dichotomy in that we have a syndrome for which there is very interesting biochemical and perhaps even autoimmune features, while the diagnosis is confirmed not by laboratory studies but on purely clinical grounds."

The most recent official definition of FS was established by a panel of experts at the Second World Congress on Myofascial Pain and Fibromyalgia, which was held in Copenhagen in August of 1992 (Kamper-Jorgensen et al. 1992). This definition states that:

> *Fibromyalgia is a painful, non-articular condition, predominantly involving muscles; it is the commonest cause of chronic, widespread musculoskeletal pain. It is typically associated with persistent fatigue, non-refreshing sleep and generalized stiffness. Women are affected some 10-20 times more often than men.*
>
> *Fibromyalgia is often part of a wider syndrome encompassing: headaches, irritable bowels, irritable bladder, dysmenorrhea, cold sensitivity, Raynaud's phenomenon, restless legs, atypical patterns of numbness and tingling, exercise intolerance, and complaints of weakness.*
>
> *A varying proportion (20-50%) of fibromyalgia patients experience significant depression or anxiety which may contribute to the severity of the symptoms or result from having chronic pain.*
>
> *Most fibromyalgia patients experience both diurnal and seasonal variations in symptoms. Typically, symptoms are worse during periods of cold damp weather, at the beginning and end of the day, and during periods of emotional stress.*

The World Health Organization has assigned fibromyalgia the number M79.0 in the International Classification of Disease (Kamper-Jorgensen et al. 1992).

Demographics

In terms of gender, women are diagnosed much more often than men. Estimates of the ratio of females to males with FS range from 4 to 20 times as many females as males. In terms of age, most patients have been diagnosed between the ages of 20 and 50 years. There seems to be an increasing number of children who are diagnosed with FS. According to many experts, only about 1% of the individuals diagnosed with FS are over the age of 60 years. However, none of the demographics have been solidly established yet.

The figures for the prevalence of FS among adults varies widely from study to study. Within some rheumatology practices, the prevalence of FS is between 13% and 20% of the clientele of those practices. Obviously, referral bias plays a part in such samplings. Dr. Wolfe (1994) recently found the prevalence among the general population to be 2%, with women making up over 90% of that group. To give some perspective to this figure, he points out that the prevalence of rheumatoid arthritis and gout is not as high as the 2% figure for FS (Wolfe 1994). This means that about five million Americans have FS, although all do not seek medical help. In terms of annual cost, it is estimated that $9.2 billion is spent each year on the treatment of individuals with FS (Russell 1994c).

In a more recent study of a random sample of 3,006 people in a community, not a clinic, 2% of the community members had FS. The diagnosis was made in accordance with the 1990 ACR criteria (see pages 10-11) (Wolfe et al. 1995). This study validates the use of the ACR criteria in the community as well as in the clinic. Interestingly, these researchers noted that the prevalence of FS actually increases with age in women. There was also an association noted between FS and divorced status and between FS and reduced family income.

Definition of Tender/Trigger Points

What is a tender point? What is a trigger point? Can the terms be used interchangeably? These terms need further clarification because the presence and status of tender points are critical for the diagnosis of fibromyalgia syndrome, according to the American College of Rheumatology (ACR) (Wolfe et al. 1990). There is consensus with the ACR criteria that a tender point is a small area in a muscle from which aching pain arises that is painful to 4 kilograms of pressure applied directly to the point. A trigger point fulfills those descriptions and, in addition, it is the source of referred pain. According to Travell and Simons (1983), there are definite and predictable referred pain patterns from each trigger point. Incidentally, Travell and Simons (1983) describe many more than the 18 tender/trigger point sites that are considered to be diagnostic by the ACR. In fact, they describe tender/trigger points in virtually every muscle in the body. Remember that the ACR has placed importance on the 18 sites that occur most frequently in fibromyalgia and the ACR has chosen to use those sites for diagnostic and research purposes. This does not mean that other trigger points should be left untreated.

Travell and Simons (1983) also differentiate between active and latent tender/trigger points. The active points are those that cause pain and usually are the motivating force behind a person seeking medical help. The latent points are those found by the examiner during the tender point site assessment. These points have not yet caused the person any pain or achiness but are painful to pressure.

Dr. Bennett (1993a) suggests that trigger or tender points "correspond to a location of insertion of muscles into ligaments or bones and are hence at a location where muscle force is transmitted through a small cross-sectional area. Tender areas often have an increased consistency compared to surrounding muscle—the so-called palpable band or fibrositic nodule."

Travell and Simons (1983, 4) contend that a trigger point is "a focus of hyperirritability in a tissue that, when compressed, is locally tender and, if sufficiently hypersensitive, gives rise to referred pain and tenderness, and sometimes to referred autonomic phenomena and distortion of proprioception." "A trigger area at a particular spot gives rise to a similar distribution of referred pain in one person as in another" which "indicates that impulses concerned in the unfamiliar reference of somatic (like visceral) pain follow fixed anatomic pathways" (Travell and Rinzler 1952, 425). This knowledge of referral patterns can help us locate a trigger point by working backward if needed. It is important to remember the inclusion of "referred autonomic phenomena and distortion of proprioception" when evaluating a client.

Travell and Simons (1983) report that trigger points are activated by overload, overwork, fatigue, direct trauma, and chilling. Trigger points (TrPs) can be indirectly activated by other trigger points, visceral disease, arthritic joints, and emotional distress. They can vary in degree of irritability from hour to hour.

Travell and Simons (1983) also note a local twitch response or transient contraction of a group of muscle fibers that harbor a trigger point when mechanically stimulated. This phenomenon is not to be confused with the jump sign, which is a general response to the pain caused by pressure on the trigger point.

Attempts at dissecting a TrP from an affected muscle have been unsuccessful as the TrP appears to be elusive. Such a concrete finding would help enormously in proving the existence of TrPs to the skeptics. However, in a recent discussion about TrPs, Dr. Travell said "she doubts that one (trigger point) will ever be discovered because she feels that it is a transitory metabolic change in muscle fibers. But whatever the reason, she gives a whole list of factors that contribute toward bringing out a TrP, such as overuse or overloading a muscle or even metabolic disease" (Colan 1994).

At present, thermography seems to offer the most objective method of identifying the locations of tender points. This instrument is able to discern temperature differences of less than one degree Centigrade. This measurement is promising because "myofascial pain typically elicits increased temperature in specific areas that are consistent with the tender points" (Hiltz 1990). Although the measurement is not absolute in its findings, it does offer some objective, machine-measured demonstration of an abnormality in the body that relates closely to tender points.

Major Associated Syndromes

Several other syndromes are frequently associated with FS, including chronic fatigue syndrome, mitral valve prolapse syndrome, irritable bowel syndrome, and Raynaud's phenomenon. It is not known whether these conditions precipitate each other or have any causal effect at all. What is known is that they tend to occur concurrently with FS. Clinically, the presence of any one of these associated syndromes can magnify the client's misery.

Chronic Fatigue Syndrome (CFS)

Some experts now consider chronic fatigue syndrome (CFS) and FS to be one entity. Research has revealed striking similarities between the two syndromes in a number of areas. In fact, 75% of people with CFS fit the criteria for a diagnosis of FS (Goldenberg et al. 1989). Chronic fatigue syndrome is ill-defined at present, with overwhelming fatigue as the diagnostic hallmark. If a person's activity level has been reduced by 50% for six months or more without an identified cause, the individual is given the diagnosis of CFS (Bennett 1990). Fatigue is a common denominator in the two syndromes, but they also share other specific details, such as similar sleep disturbances (Whelton, Salit, and Moldofsky 1992), and low natural killer (NK) cell activity (Komaroff and Buchwald 1991). These findings have given rise to the idea that CFS and FS may be the same syndrome or at least on the same spectrum. Supporting this idea is the following statement in which one could easily substitute "fibromyalgia syndrome" each time "chronic fatigue syndrome" is named.

> *Despite preliminary data, no physical finding or laboratory test was deemed confirmatory of the diagnosis of chronic fatigue syndrome. For assessment of clinical status, investigators must rely on the use of standardized instruments for patient self-reporting of fatigue, mood disturbance, functional status, sleep disorder, global well-being, and pain. Further research is needed to develop better instruments for quantifying these domains in patients with chronic fatigue syndrome* (Schluerderberg et al. 1992).

For awhile, CFS was thought to be caused by a virus, the best known of which was the Epstein-Barr virus. Seemingly, this drew a distinction between CFS and FS; however, this idea has been disproved. Dr. Stephen Straus elaborates on the topic of a viral etiology pointing out that most of such research has yielded unclear or weak conclusions despite the widely read *Newsweek* article (published mid-1980s) that convinced many people that Epstein-Barr virus was the culprit in CFS (Straus 1994). There are some cases of CFS, as well as some cases of FS, that seem to have been triggered by a virus. But most cases of both syndromes clearly were not induced by a virus. In discussing this controversy, Dr. I. Jon Russell has pointed out that in his practice he has not seen patients with FS who have tender lymph nodes or recurrent fevers. Nor does he see spouses of patients with FS who also have FS, but he does see spouses of CFS patients who also have CFS (Straus 1994). There are still a number of differences that have not yet been reconciled, which prevents consensus on this matter at present. Therefore, for the purposes of this manual, FS will be treated as a separate entity from CFS.

Mitral Valve Prolapse Syndrome (MVP)

A condition very commonly found in people with FS is mitral valve prolapse syndrome (MVP). The prolapse happens in the mitral valve of the heart when part of the valve that connects the left atrium and the left ventricle does not close tightly. This is usually due to a malformation of one of the leaflets of the valve. When the left ventricle contracts, the pressure pushes against the faulty valve and part of it flutters back up into the atrium. The diagnosis may be suspected during the course of a physical exam because the examiner will note a characteristic clicking sound. An echocardiogram is necessary to confirm the diagnosis. Even with this high-technology exam, a false negative is possible. This has also been called Barlow's syndrome, floppy valve syndrome, click-murmur syndrome, and a benign murmur. Pellegrino and colleagues (1989) found that the incidence of MVP among people with FS was 75%, whereas it is only 5% to 17% among the general population.

A syndrome has been delineated to encompass a host of symptoms often encountered by people who have mitral valve prolapse. The mitral valve prolapse syndrome, which has been described in *Confronting Mitral Valve Prolapse Syndrome* (Frederickson 1988), shares many characteristics with the fibromyalgia syndrome, including sleep disturbance, fatigue, female predominance, exercise intolerance, and anxiety. Indeed, panic attacks are common in people with MVP syndrome.

Of special interest regarding people with MVP syndrome is the feature called dysautonomia. This label reflects a disturbance in the autonomic nervous system and seems to explain most of the symptoms, such as fatigue, anxiety, and hyper-vigilance, according to Frederickson (1988). The author also suggests that the relationship between the mitral valve and the autonomic nervous system begins very early as they are both formed at the same embryonic stage. She points out that an imbalance could occur either because the sympathetic nervous system becomes overactive or because the parasympathetic nervous system becomes less active than normal. Such an imbalance seems to be a major factor in FS also but it has not been called dysautonomia in the FS literature. In treating dysautonomia in the MVP syndrome population, Frederickson states that the offending system can be identified using noninvasive testing and the patient can be medicated accordingly. Frederickson points out that this type of dysautonomia is not the same as that caused by damaged nerves which occurs in people with diabetes and coronary heart disease.

Irritable Bowel Syndrome (IBS)

Many people with FS experience a disturbance in their bowel function that has been labeled irritable bowel syndrome (previously known as spastic colon or nervous stomach). The problem is bewildering as diarrhea and constipation may alternate within a short time frame and abdominal pain is often severe. It has been suggested by I. Jon Russell, M.D., that the reduced level of serotonin and increased level of substance P probably have an effect on bowel motility and homeostasis (Russell 1994b). Apparently, both serotonin and substance P normally appear in the intestinal tract when digestion begins. Not much is known about the digestive functions of these chemicals. To understand the possible connection of serotonin to IBS, a chapter in the *Handbook of Experimental Pharmacology* (Erspamer 1966) offers some answers. According to Erspamer, some serotonin is manufactured outside the brain and occurs primarily in the enterochromaffin cells of the intestines. Platelet vesicles then become the storage house for this serotonin. The platelet membranes have a re-uptake receptor for serotonin by which the platelets collect the serotonin. The density of these receptor sites was studied by Russell and colleagues (1992a). Surprisingly, individuals with FS had a greater density of receptor sites than the control group. The suggestion for rationalization of these findings is that the increase of receptor sites may be a response to a decrease in the amount of serotonin in the blood. If this rationalization is correct, then it represents an example of the body attempting to reestablish homeostasis. Perhaps this disturbance in the balance of the serotonin mechanism contributes to the problems associated with irritable bowel syndrome.

Raynaud's Phenomenon

Another commonly associated syndrome is Raynaud's phenomenon or Raynaud's syndrome. Vaerøy and colleagues (1988) define this condition as "(a) a triphasic color response where pallor, cyanosis and rubor appear in that sequence; (b) a vasospastic disorder with intermittent attacks of ischemia mainly in the fingers and toes; and (c) known to be triggered by cold or emotional stimuli and is often accompanied by paresthesia and pain." In their study, the researchers found that 53% of people with FS had Raynaud's syndrome or Raynaud's-like symptoms. In the same study, the level of substance P in the subjects' cerebrospinal fluid was found to be elevated in people with FS but the substance P level did not correlate with the incidence or severity of the Raynaud's-like symptoms, implying that substance P might have little impact on Raynaud's phenomenon. In a follow-up study, Vaerøy and colleagues (1989) studied Raynaud's and substance P and demonstrated that less vasoconstriction occurred in the hands of individuals with FS. This finding was unexpected because the study subjects had all indicated that they did, indeed, have Raynaud's syndrome. One explanation offered by the authors is that the subjects actually experienced hyperactivity of the sympathetic nervous system and that there might have been an exhaustion of the system.

Lyme Disease

FS and CFS have been reported as frequent sequelae or concomitant developments to Lyme disease. In fact, FS/CFS is considered the worst complication of Lyme disease (Steere et al. 1993). In 15 cases of Lyme disease-related fibromyalgia, repeated courses of antibiotics aimed at B. burgdorferi (the spirochete that causes Lyme disease) are ineffective in relieving the FS symptoms (Dinerman and Steere 1992). The authors suggest that B. burgdorferi may trigger the onset of FS.

Human Immunodeficiency Virus (HIV)

Among people infected with HIV, FS is the most prevalent musculoskeletal complication. It has been reported by Buskila and colleagues (1990) to occur in as many as 20% of people with HIV. It has also been noted by Simms and colleagues (1992) that HIV patients who have FS experience worse depression than HIV patients without FS.

Other Associated Conditions

There have also been some cases of the onset of FS following an infection of coxsackie (Nash, Chard, and Hagleman 1989) as well as the parvovirus (Leventhal, Naides, and Freundlich 1991). However, it is atypical to find serologic evidence of parvovirus infection in people with FS (Leventhal, Naides, and Freundlich 1991). There are several seeming paradoxes in the fibromyalgia syndrome. We see one of them in this discussion of associated syndromes. Infection appears to have some sort of causal (or triggering) relationship to FS, yet research and lab work do not strongly support this notion. Dr. Goldenberg (1994b) suggests that there are two approaches to sorting out this paradox. One is the classic medical model of such a relationship in which an infectious agent would invade body tissues and/or activate cytokines and other immune mediators. This would be a directly causal relationship and we would expect to find evidence of an infectious agent in the tissues or central nervous system of the patient. According to Dr. Goldenberg, there is no such evidence. In the classic medical model, antibiotic treatment in Lyme disease-associated fibromyalgia would be beneficial. However, this has not been the case. Therefore, the classic medical model does not seem to be helpful in explaining the findings. The other approach that Dr. Goldenberg suggests involves the fact "that infections precipitate a negative adaptation to stress which is then responsible for the chronic symptoms. In such a model, infections may be one of many stressors that lead to avoidance behavior, mood, and sleep disturbances, muscle tension, and diminished exercise capacity" (Goldenberg 1994b, 54).

Overview of FS Research Findings

As medical professionals who work with patients with musculoskeletal pain, it is important to explore the treatment possibilities that research is providing. We have an obligation to seek more knowledge so that we can better serve our clients and our profession. In the words of Dr. I. Jon Russell (1993a), "Pain is a symptom which has been difficult to confirm and to quantify but that does not excuse the medical community from developing new methods for doing so. Most of the pain experienced by patients has a physiological or biochemical explanation. It is not the patient's responsibility to change her disease into something we know more about. Rather, it is our task to better understand the problem she has."

A review of some of the research findings provides an increased understanding of the mysteries and the complexities of FS. Categorizing the research helps to make it clearer. It is impossible to do this in a strict manner because the syndrome affects many parts of the body and is affected by a variety of stimuli. The interactions of chemicals, tissues, and systems are continuous and intertwined. Generally speaking, there have been two approaches to research: studies that targeted peripheral structures as the "end organ," such as the muscle or nerves, and studies that investigated some central mechanism, such as neurotransmitters or misinterpretation of pain signals. Keep in mind that the divisions between these categories are insubstantial. Much of the research crosses these divisions effortlessly.

Many research projects have been published in which intriguing information has been learned about the biochemistry, neurological functions, and reactions of species other than humans. These may help enlighten us regarding the mysteries of FS; however, in this manual, studies using other species have been omitted except for a few cases. For the most part, the studies that have involved humans are the focus.

For the sake of organization, research that has focused on muscle or muscle membrane defects, microcirculation disturbance, and responses to exercise are categorized under the heading Peripheral Mechanisms. Research on neurotransmitters, infectious processes, the hypothalamus-pituitary-adrenal axis, environmental sensitivities, immunological reactions, psychological status, medications, and nutrition are considered Central Mechanisms.

Peripheral Mechanisms
Muscle and Muscle Membrane Damage

In recognition of the fact that muscle pain is often the symptom that provokes a fibromyalgia syndrome (FS) sufferer to seek medical attention, investigation of affected muscle tissue is a logical approach for research. Muscle pain is also one of the chief diagnostic criteria of the syndrome. Several researchers have studied possible focal changes in muscle and they have uncovered some significant features of fibromyalgic muscle tissue. For instance, Robert Bennett, M.D., of Oregon Health Sciences University in Portland has developed a model of muscle micro-trauma as a cause of the muscle pain in FS (Bennett 1993a).

Microtrauma can be caused by a one-time trauma, such as an accident, or by re-petitive insults, such as maintaining one position to perform a job every day. Dr. Bennett thinks eccentric muscle contractions could also cause microtrauma. He postulates that microtrauma to the muscle causes a breakdown of the sarcolemmal membrane. When this barrier between the muscle fiber and the extracellular fluid has been compromised, calcium ions flood into the muscle fiber. This influx of calcium ions activates other reactions, which ultimately produce free oxygen rad-icals, according to the work of Jackson, Jones, and Edwards (1984). These chem-icals then launch an attack on the sarcolemmal membrane. Thus, the effects of the original microtrauma may be perpetuated. To make matters worse for the damaged sarcolemmal membrane, individuals with FS apparently produce a reduced level of growth hormone, which is a vital part of the process of cell membrane repair (Bennett 1993a).

Another aspect of Dr. Bennett's model is that the influx of calcium ions results in what Dr. Bennett calls a "nonphysiological contraction" of the involved sarco-meres. This is a very important point in trying to understand the nature of the focal tenderness found in people with FS. Other researchers suggest that this type of focal event in adjoining sarcomeres accounts for the phenomenon called taut bands (Jacobsen, Bartels, and Danneskiold-Samsøe 1991). These focal nonphysiological contractions could also account for the restricted range of motion that is often seen in individuals with FS. Dr. Bennett takes his hypothesis a step further to explain another typical complaint, muscle stiffness. He hypothesizes that the muscle spin-dles take their cues from this restricted range of motion and then they reset the dynamic tension of the muscle (Bennett 1993a). As the muscle spindles reset, the muscle fibers accept a tighter setting as the new resting state when, in fact, those fibers are not at rest at all. This manifests itself as "stiffness."

Yet another aspect of Dr. Bennett's model deals with adenosine triphosphate (ATP). When the calcium ions flood into the muscle fiber, the calcium pumps work hard to re-establish the correct balance in the fiber. Apparently these pumps are fueled by ATP and the flurry of activity leads to a fuel shortage. This leaves the muscle fiber with an energy crisis due to below-normal levels of ATP. Supporting this model is a study done in 1986 that indicated a reduced level of ATP in fibromyalgic muscles as well as evidence of ragged-red muscle fibers at the sites of tenderness (Bengtsson, Henriksson, and Larsson 1986a).

On the other hand, Nørregaard and colleagues (1994a) conducted a study of cell morphology in people with FS and found no difference in the ATP or the ADP content of muscles. However, the biopsies they used were taken from the vastus lateralis muscle and were not taken at a tender point site as had been done in the previous studies in which alteration in the high-energy phosphate levels had been reported.

Why does microtrauma lead to this chain of events in some people but not in others? Dr. Bennett suggests a polygenic inheritance pattern for such vulnerability (Bennett 1993a). He feels that some other factors must be present in combination with a genetic predisposition in order for the syndrome to manifest. In fact, his suggestion has been supported by the research done by Pellegrino, Waylonis, and Sommer (1989) in which they documented a familial tendency to the development of fibromyalgia.

Another approach to the study of the peripheral theory of the cause of FS has been provided by researchers who use electromyography (EMG) studies to elucidate the condition of the fibromyalgic muscle. Zidar and colleagues (1990) performed EMGs of the painful muscles of people with FS and found no detectable abnormality. Their conclusion was that this lack of EMG abnormality indicates that there must be some other source of pain than the muscle fiber itself. On the other hand, some researchers have reported EMG changes in their studies. For instance, Hubbard and Berkoff (1993) found that when the needle was inserted into the 1 to 2 millimeter nidus of a tender point at a depth of about 2 centimeters, activity was noted in all subjects. They report that the activity was maintained as long as the needle was in place. The maximum amount of time tested was 50 minutes. Movement of the needle away from the nidus by as little as 1 millimeter caused a cessation of the EMG activity. This spontaneous EMG activity correlated with an increase of symptoms of pain, radiating pain, and autonomic responses such as nausea and excessive sweating. Hubbard and Berkoff theorize that the intrafusal fibers of the muscle spindle become overstimulated by an overactive sympathetic nervous system. This overstimulated state sets up a chronic low-grade muscle tension that may cause pain.

Muscle biopsy is an obvious way to determine differences in muscle tissues. What have muscle biopsy studies revealed about fibromyalgic muscles? So far this has been a disappointing avenue for understanding FS. An early study showed ragged red fibers, which indicate metabolic distress, but recent studies show little more than type 2 atrophy, which can be attributed to disuse (Bengtsson, Henriksson, and Larsson 1986b). In all the biopsy research that has been done, little evidence of inflammation has been found (Kalyan-Raman et al. 1984; Schroder, Drewes, and Andreasen 1993). As a result, the accepted name for this syndrome was changed from *fibrositis* to *fibromyalgia*.

Microcirculation Compromise

Yet another possible peripheral culprit is microcirculation, which would result in tissue hypoxia. To determine the oxygenation of muscle tissue in which tender/trigger points are found, a study was performed in Sweden utilizing the MDO oxygen electrode (Lund, Bengtsson, and Thorborg 1986). The researchers tested the trapezius and brachioradialis muscles of people with FS and compared them to a control group. At each site, the oxygen pressure was measured at eight points simultaneously. In order to allow for the continual alterations in tissue oxygenation, measurements at each site were recorded every 15 seconds for 2 minutes. Abnormal oxygenation in these muscles was found. However, Sietsema and colleagues (1993) also studied the possibility of muscle ischemia and their measurements did not reveal any abnormality in tissue oxygenation. An interesting note to their study was that it was impossible to obtain maximal exercise from the FS group due to pain.

If the microcirculation is compromised and causes hypoxia in the surrounding tissues, ATP production will also be compromised due to a decrease in the amount of available oxygen. It is suggested by Mense and Stahnke (1983) that hypoxia in a muscle that is trying to do work can irritate pain receptors. This may happen via algogenic substances that tend to build up in the presence of hypoxia. The ATP stored in the muscle is used within a few seconds. This means that a fresh supply is needed on a constant basis. But oxygen is needed to produce more ATP. When the balance tips to the side of hypoxia and low ATP production, pain is the result, according to Henriksson (1993). He suggests that a localized microcirculatory disturbance could thus account for the fibromyalgia pain during activity. Work by Lewis, Pickering, and Rothschild (1931) on intermittent claudication corroborates the basic concept that pain will develop in a muscle that is contracting in an ischemic environment. They report that muscle pain will ensue within one minute under those conditions.

Several suggestions have been made regarding the mechanism involved in creating the muscle pain. One of the most common ideas offered is that lactic acid buildup causes the pain. Musculoskeletal research on patients who have McArdle's disease (myophosphorylase deficiency) indicates that this is not necessarily the answer. McArdle's disease is a condition in which the individuals affected are unable to use muscle glycogen for energy and, as a result, do not produce lactic acid (Rodbard 1975). Even so, these patients do experience muscle pain. This finding casts doubt on lactic acid buildup as the culprit in the muscle pain of people with FS. At least it allows for some other possibility.

On the other hand, research by Wagenmakers, Coakley, and Edwards (1988) in England has shown that deconditioned muscles have a decreased concentration of mitochondria. Individuals with such a condition apparently tend to overutilize glycolysis, which leads to an increased level of lactate being produced. This occurs even with low-intensity exercise. It is suggested that the amount of exercise that can be done without excessive glycolysis is set by the concentration of mitochondria in the type II fibers that have the lowest capacity for aerobic metabolism when the muscle is untrained. The proportion of these type II fibers increases with a decrease in activity by the muscle. As this occurs, a new limit is set for the amount of exercise possible without lactate production. Thus, a cycle emerges.

The pain that most people with FS experience when they are at rest is still unexplained. A study by Backman and colleagues (1988) indicates that a reduced relaxation rate may be part of the answer. The results of an EMG study by Elert and colleagues (1992) seem to relate to Backman's study. These researchers found insufficient relaxation between contractions in all the shoulder girdle muscles of the FS subjects. Henriksson (1993) theorizes that "static work and deficient relaxation over long periods of time are possible factors. Some motor units may be active more or less continuously both during static and dynamic muscular contractions. Postischemic damage is another possibility." Interestingly, regional sympathetic (stellate ganglion) blocks have been shown to relieve pain at rest and to reduce the number of tender points (Bengtsson and Bengtsson 1988). This finding points to an etiology in the autonomic nervous system.

Exercise

Exercise is currently one of the most widely accepted tools for alleviating the symptoms of FS. What we know from research about the effect of exercise on FS can guide our use of exercise in treating people with FS.

A controlled study of the aerobic fitness of people with FS showed that 80% of the subjects were aerobically unfit. The subjects exercised on a bicycle ergometer to exhaustion. Maximal oxygen uptake was used to determine aerobic fitness. Also, the clearance of 133 xenon from the blood of exercising muscles was measured and noted to be significantly poorer in people with FS than in the control group. The assumption was made that becoming aerobically fit would benefit individuals with FS (Bennett et al. 1989). In another study involving aerobic exercise, 51 people were divided into three groups and treated either with amitriptyline (a medication in the tricyclic family), cardiovascular training, or a combination of the two for 15 weeks. Only the combination group improved in terms of pain tolerance in the tender points, which was determined with the use of a dolorimeter (Isomeri et al. 1993).

McCain and colleagues (1988) studied 42 patients for 20 weeks. These subjects either participated in a cardiovascular fitness training program or a flexibility training program. The researchers found that aerobic fitness increased in 83% of the people in the cardiovascular fitness training program, but in only one person in the flexibility training group. Objective and subjective measurements of pain indicated that the subjects in the cardiovascular fitness training group had improved in terms of their level of pain. Curiously, there was no change in the amount of disturbed sleep in either group.

Another study demonstrated that sleep deprivation led to FS-like pain even among healthy subjects. However, the subjects who were affected least by the sleep deprivation were those who were aerobically fit (Moldofsky et al. 1975).

These studies support the assumption that cardiovascular training is beneficial for individuals with FS. However, the client with FS is often unhappy to be told that exercise is important in managing this condition and relates instances of feeling worse following exercise. If exercise is considered to be one of our most important tools for managing fibromyalgia, then we must figure out how to fine tune our approach so that the patient does not feel worse from using this tool.

One aspect of this fine tuning includes modifying the level of intensity of the exercise regime. Research by Mengshoel and Førre (1993) found that people with FS can perform low-intensity exercises without exacerbation of pain and fatigue. Two groups of people with FS were followed over a period of 20 weeks. One group did not change their physical activity level. The other group added one hour of exercise two times per week to their normal level of physical activity. The exercise group participated in a modified, low-impact aerobic dance program in which the heart rate did not exceed 150 beats per minute. After the exercise, 100% reported a feeling of well-being and nine patients in the exercise group reported less muscle tension. However, there was no significant change in pain and fatigue levels reported among the exercise group.

Another study was designed to explore the possibility that certain chemicals developed during or after exercise might cause the muscle pain complained of by people with FS (Nørregaard, et al. 1994a). Nørregaard and colleagues measured lactate and potassium during a bicycle ergometer test and found that, overall, these were similar between people with FS and the control group. However, among the group with FS, there were significantly higher levels of lactate at mid-range of the workload. They also measured plasma creatine kinase and myoglobin at 45 minutes one day and two days after the exercise test. The hematocrit was similar between the two groups and the plasma creatine kinase was significantly higher in the group with FS 45 minutes after the test. After one and two days, the measurements were similar; yet the perceived pain using a visual analogue scale increased from 30% prior to exercise to 86% on the first day after exercise and 78% on the second day after exercise. The researchers concluded that the pain-causing mechanism is not in the parameter they studied but is likely to be found in an altered central mechanism, or the pain may occur in the tendons or ligaments rather than the muscle fibers.

To find out whether people with FS accurately perceive their level of exertion during exercise, 95 women with FS were tested. Oxygen consumption and carbon dioxide production were measured while each subject walked on a treadmill. Heart rate, workload, minutes of exercise, and the subject's rating of perceived exertion were recorded. Fifty percent of the subjects appropriately perceived their level of exertion and 34% overestimated it. The results suggest that most people with FS do rate their exertion level correctly (Clark et al. 1993).

Several researchers have found abnormal responses to exercise in people with FS. In one such study, the patients were asked to exercise on a bicycle ergometer. Measurements of ACTH and cortisol were made at intervals (Griep, Boersma, and deKloet 1993). There was an abnormally high release of ACTH early in the exercise test at submaximal levels though no corresponding elevation of cortisol occurred. Exercise of 50 to 80 watts does not normally cause any increase in ACTH or cortisol (Few 1974). After exhaustion was reached, people with FS had higher ACTH and cortisol levels than the control group. This indicates involvement of the hypothalamus-pituitary-adrenal axis, which leads researchers to theorize that people with FS suffer from pain and fatigue (stressors). It is the pain and fatigue that account for the abnormal responses rather than the effort of the exercise, according to this finding. Other researchers have supported this stress-due-to-pain theory in their work (Lundberg and Frankenhaeuser 1980).

Dr. Goldstein (1993b) also tested the response of people with FS to exercising on a bicycle ergometer. He used a SPECT scan and measured cerebral blood flow as well as temperature, cortisol production, growth hormone production, and catecholamine (norepinephrine and epinephrine) level after exercise. In healthy people, all of these parameters typically increase in response to exercise, but in the group with FS, there were no increases of these parameters and the temperature and cerebral blood flow actually decreased. A similar study was done in the Netherlands with confirming results (van Denderen et al. 1992). The subjects and controls exercised vigorously using a bicycle ergometer and steps. Levels of serum creatine kinase, myoglobin, cortisol, epinephrine, and norepinephrine were measured and all were reduced in the group with FS. The findings, while striking, can be explained by a decreased hypothalamic-pituitary-adrenal axis response, a diminished sympathetic nervous system response, or a combination of the two. These results might even be caused by a reduced amount of work delivered by the FS group. The researchers also found lower heart rates in the FS group and this, apparently, implies subdued sympathetic reactivity.

Dr. Bennett (1993b) used NMR spectroscopy to investigate the muscles of 11 people with FS and 10 sedentary controls following fatiguing exercise. All of the individuals with FS showed abnormality of phospho-diester compounds compared to only 50% of the controls. He suggests that this is caused by muscle membrane damage. This is consistent with the fact that people with FS also have decreased growth hormone production and, consequently, poor repair of the muscles and membranes.

Dr. Moldofsky (1993) conducted a study recently on the chronobiology of FS, which revealed that people with FS feel best between 10:00 a.m. and 2:00 p.m. He suggested that people with FS exercise during that time period. In an Australian study on the diurnal variation of FS symptoms, tender points were tested with a dolorimeter in the morning and evening. Tender points were more numerous and more painful in the evening (Reilly and Littlejohn 1993b). Unfortunately, dolorimeter examinations were not performed at mid-day, but subjects reported feeling best at mid-day.

Weltman and DeVries and their colleagues showed in separate studies that healthy people produce an increased amount of growth hormone as a result of exercise (Weltman et al. 1992; DeVries et al. 1991). These results are the underlying rationale for using exercise to manage fibromyalgia syndrome because it is known that people with FS have abnormally low levels of growth hormone in their bodies. It is assumed that people with FS will respond to exercise as healthy people do in terms of increased growth hormone production. Increased growth hormone would induce greater production of insulin-like growth factor by the liver. "One of the tasks given to insulin-like growth factor is to maintain the health of skeletal muscle" (Russell 1994d, 79).

It has been noted by many researchers and clinicians that most people with FS are deconditioned, seemingly due to their intolerance of exercise. Simms (1994) felt that many of the studies had failed to match the subjects of the study with deconditioned controls. Also, the muscles studied in these cases were often muscles that do not commonly contain tender points. Therefore, he performed a study that matched subjects and controls for deconditioning. He also chose to study one muscle that typically contains tender points for people with FS (the upper trapezius) and one muscle that does not (the tibialis anterior) using phosphate nuclear magnetic resonance spectroscopy. He described this method as "a non-invasive approach to measure important metabolites in muscle energy metabolism such as phosphocreatine (PCr), inorganic phosphate (Pi), adenosine triphosphate (ATP), and intracellular muscle pH" (Simms 1994, 118). Using isometric contractions, he found that the levels of maximum oxygen uptake, phosphocreatine, inorganic phosphate, and intracellular pH were similar between the group with FS and the control group. The isometric muscle strength was also similar between the two groups. Simms suggests that the pain associated with FS might be better explained by a central mechanism since he found no abnormalities in the peripheral factors that he studied.

In another experiment, researchers concluded that it may be erroneous to blame poor fitness levels in people with FS for the poor physical performance they exhibit. In fact, it appears that some of the blame may rest with the muscle soreness that they experience (Verstapen et al. 1995). In other words, these individuals often stop a physical test early because of muscle soreness, thereby leaving their true fitness level to guesswork. People with FS tended to withhold their maximum effort on subsequent tests if they had experienced muscle soreness during one of the fitness tests. Interestingly, the researchers found that the people with FS who had previously been more athletic exhibited higher levels on the fitness tests than did those with FS who had never been physically active. This study consisted of 12 fitness tests in which 87 FS patients were matched with healthy controls.

Nørregaard, Bülow, and Danneskiold-Samsøe (1994) investigated the decreased muscle strength and endurance that are characteristic of people with FS to determine whether inactivity could account for these complaints. The subjects of study were age- and sex-matched with a sedentary control group. The group with FS measured 30% to 40% weaker per cross-sectional area in the voluntary muscle strength of the quadriceps muscle. The researchers suggested that this finding supports a strength training aspect for the treatment of people with FS. They concluded that this deficiency in muscle strength could be explained either by physical inactivity and/or neuroendocrine factors.

Klug, McAuley, and Clark (1989) studied the changes that occur in the trained muscles when unilateral training (riding a stationary bicycle with one leg) is used. They found that "the activity of the mitochondrial marker enzyme succinate dehydrogenase was significantly elevated in the trained leg" (p. 33). They also noted that the muscle metabolism shifted to utilization of fats in the trained leg. This seems to imply that training can be helpful in weight control. Often people with FS complain that they have gained weight since they have become less active in response to their aversion to exercise.

Central Mechanisms

Immune System and Limbic System

The significance of impairments in the immune system in relationship to FS has recently been identified and has inspired increasing interest and research in the last few years. Because FS patients do not exhibit characteristics that are immediately reminiscent of autoimmune diseases, this area of research was slow to develop. Now we can expect to see an explosion of information resulting from new research.

Research published by Xavier Caro, M.D. (1984), pointed out the presence of immune reactive proteins in the skin of 76% of the people with FS who were studied. Normally these immune reactive proteins are not found in skin. This finding suggests the likelihood of an immunologic aspect of FS because proteins are known to move through the walls of blood vessels in other immunologically related conditions.

Another immunological clue is the elevated level of interleukin-2 that occurred in 12 people with FS, which points to the presence of an infectious process in that the immune system produces this cytokine to fight infection (Hader 1994).

Yet another immunological puzzle piece involves the natural killer cells. Natural killer cells are a specific type of lymphocyte that select and kill certain tumor cells, microorganisms, and cells infected by viruses (Mackinnon 1989). The level of activity of natural killer cells has been found to be low in individuals with FS by I. Jon Russell, M.D., and colleagues (1988) and, in an independent study, by X. Caro, M.D. (1994).

Obviously, it is impossible to completely isolate a system of the human body. All of the systems overlap and interact. This is certainly evident in discussing the research on FS. The work of Dr. Moldofsky and colleagues (1986, 1989) of Toronto regarding the influences that sleep and the immune system have on each other is an example of research that overlaps several areas. He showed that sleep deprivation causes alterations in the levels of interleukin-1 (IL-1) and interleukin-2 (IL-2) (cytokines) and natural killer cell activity. Conversely, he showed that changes in IL-1 and IL-2 cause changes in the sleep architecture. Dr. Moldofsky (1992) states that individuals with FS often demonstrate elevated levels of these two cytokines. This abnormal state can cause muscular pain, fatigue, and memory dysfunction.

Some people trace the onset of their FS symptoms to a severe bout with influenza. What could be the relationship? The responsible agent may be the muramyl dipeptides that are released from cell walls of friendly bacteria when the bacteria are digested in the stomach. This is a normal process. These dipeptides travel through the blood and activate serotonin receptors in the brain. Because of this activity, these dipeptides become an important link in normal serotonin function. (The importance of normal serotonin function to the sleep-wake cycle and to FS are discussed on pages 38 to 40.) If the normal cycle of friendly bacteria digestion is interrupted by an infectious agent, then the chain of events leading to deep sleep will likely be disrupted also. To further disrupt this process, the antibiotic medicines prescribed for influenza often decimate the friendly bacteria population while fighting the infectious agents, which leaves the person free of the infection but vulnerable to the problems associated with sleep disruption (Caro 1994).

Another aspect of the infectious agent theory of etiology is that the process of fighting the infectious agent requires high use of energy compounds such as adenosine triphosphate (ATP) and nicotinamide adenine dinucleotide phosphate (NADP). The invader eventually leaves, but the damage to the immune system may be long-lasting, according to Mark Loveless, M.D. (1994). In fact, the infectious agent may be the triggering event for people who have a genetic predisposition to developing FS.

A slightly different twist to this trigger theory is that a flu-like syndrome can occur due to exposure to chemicals that are toxic to the individual. Gunnar Heuser, M.D., Ph.D. (1993), believes this vulnerable situation can encourage the development of an actual infectious process (Heuser 1993). This vulnerable state can be caused by simply smelling a toxic chemical. For individuals who are chemically sensitive, chemicals that are found in everyday household items may be toxic to them. The triggering chemicals seem to vary, but common offenders include the petroleum-based products in new carpeting and new upholstery. According to Dr. Heuser, "Toxic chemical exposure often causes a flu-like syndrome which includes headaches, muscle aches and pains, night sweats, and a sore throat. In addition, impairment of brain function (especially memory) and chronic fatigue frequently develop. Finally, infections (viral, bacterial, fungal) and multiple chemical sensitivities often ensue. In severe cases, disability is seen" (Heuser 1993).

Iris Bell, M.D., Ph.D. (1993), suggests that the explanation for chemical sensitivity is to be found in the limbic system of the brain because the olfactory system is the direct pathway to the limbic system. There is no blood-brain barrier to toxic odors, which means that these toxic odors are not filtered out. As a result, instead of the effect of the chemicals being modulated, the effect might actually be amplified.

The limbic system is a major regulatory agency in the brain and it is anatomically situated so that it can be a link between various areas of the brain and the neuro-endocrine system. Are there other connections between the limbic system and FS? A number of researchers have been helping to answer that question. Dr. Goldstein (1993a, 10) has stated that,

> *The limbic system is a high-order regulatory part of the brain that works somewhat like a computer to integrate input and determine the appropriate response for a given situation. It seems to me that the 'computer' or limbic system isn't working right in CFS and FS patients. It is too sensitive to certain stimuli, it doesn't filter them out properly (through a mechanism called sensory gating). And it doesn't process the inputs correctly either . . . The limbic system forms a ring around the center of the brain and has projections to virtually all of the areas in the central nervous system.*

One of the limbic system's functions is to regulate some of the stress responses of the body. Dr. Goldstein (1993b) asked patients to ride an exercise bike to exhaustion and then took five measurements. He measured temperature, cortisol production, growth hormone production, catecholamine level, and cerebral blood flow. In a normal population, an increase in all of these measurements would be seen. In people with FS and CFS, none of the measurements increased and temperature and cerebral blood flow actually decreased. Dr. Goldstein takes these findings as evidence that there could be a dysfunction in the limbic system in response to stress.

In the Netherlands, other researchers found that cortisol levels in individuals with FS were decreased after exhausting exercise (van Denderen et al. 1992). They also proposed the possibility that this result might reflect a disturbance in the hypothalamic-pituitary-adrenal axis in response to chronic stress.

Anatomically connected with the limbic system is the caudate nucleus, which is thought to be involved in memory and concentration tasks as well as pain regulation. Using SPECT scans, Drs. Mountz and Bradley (1994) found decreased blood flow in the caudate nuclei in people with FS. (Apparently, individuals with reflex sympathetic dystrophy show a similar abnormality.) The amount of abnormality in the blood flow correlated directly with the pain scores of the subjects with FS.

With regard to abnormal blood flow in the brain, Dr. Romano (1994) studied 100 people with FS who had headaches. He also found abnormalities on SPECT scans. Ninety-seven percent of the subjects studied showed a difference in blood flow between the right and left hemispheres of the brain. In most cases, the difference noted was a reduction in flow in the temporal or frontal lobe areas. He concluded that some of the medications currently used for vascular headaches might be useful for FS patients who suffer headaches frequently.

People with FS often exhibit a hypersensitive or hypervigilant state in relation to their environment. Many people with FS describe situations in which their bodies react in a hyperactive way. For example, when other people simply notice a strong odor, such as a new carpet, some people with FS will associate the onset of nausea, headache, or other pain with the smell. Another example is the typical complaint of being a light sleeper, a characteristic that has also been termed "hypervigilant." This term may also be applied to an individual who experiences prolonged "fight or flight" stimulation and whose sympathetic nervous system remains over-stimulated perpetually.

Gerster and Hadj-Djilani (1984) found that FS symptoms may be precipitated by loud noises. Because noise intolerance has also been observed in people treated with tricyclics, all of the research subjects had to be free of these drugs for at least one month prior to the study. Twenty percent of the group with FS developed muscle pain secondary to the loud noise, while 70% exhibited a diminished painful sound threshold (PST). The PST occurred below 100 decibels hearing level (dBHL) at all frequencies for both ears in the group with FS. The control group still had PSTs of at least 110 dBHL. Forty percent of the group with FS also exhibited increased vestibular excitability, which indicates a central nervous system prob-lem. Apparently this can occur when there is increased tone in the cervical muscles as well as when a person is overly anxious. (Both of these symptoms occur in individuals with FS.) None of the abnormalities could be explained by physical examination as no physical abnormalities were noted.

Sensitivity of people with FS to thermal pain was demonstrated by Gibson and colleagues (1994). The researchers tested subjects on the dorsum of the hand and over certain tender point sites using carbon dioxide laser stimulation and found that the group with FS had a significantly lower heat pain threshold than the control group. They took the study one step further and noted that the individuals who experienced the largest flare response (pain) were the ones who also displayed the greatest reduction in pain threshold. The researchers also confirmed previous work showing that people with FS have a lower mechanical pain threshold as well. They measured the cerebral potentials evoked by the carbon dioxide stimulation and thereby found significant evidence of increased activation of the central nervous system (CNS) among the group with FS. These potentials were called nociceptive evoked responses (NERs) and the amplitude of the NERs was nearly double that of the control group. This finding is considered to be evidence that people with FS "exhibit a marked increase in the CNS response to incoming nociceptive input" (Gibson et al. 1994, 191).

Responses to Stress: Hypothalamus-Pituitary-Adrenal Axis and the Autonomic Nervous System

The stress system of the body is very complex and involves several components. Two of the major components are the hypothalamus-pituitary-adrenal axis and the locus ceruleus-norepinephrine/autonomic (sympathetic) systems. Adaptational re-sponses to stressors can be dealt with via these systems. "Generally, the stress response is meant to be acute or at least of a limited duration. The time-limited nature of this process renders its accompanying antianabolic, catabolic, and im-munosuppressive effects temporarily beneficial and of no adverse consequences" (Chrousos and Gold 1992, 1247). Chrousos and Gold discuss the negative effects of a chronic or excessive activation of the stress response, which seems to cause a number of disease states and may account for some of the problems associated with FS.

The first component of the stress system involves the interactions of the hypothalamus, the pituitary gland, the adrenal gland, and the hypothalamus-pituitary-adrenal axis (HPA). On a chemical level, the adaptational response is modulated significantly by corticotropin-releasing hormone (CRH) synthesis and its release, which occurs primarily in the paraventricular nucleus of the hypothalamus (Chrousos and Gold 1992). Several factors can influence the production of CRH, including serotonin, pointing out again the importance of serotonin.

CRH causes the release of adrenocorticotropin hormone (ACTH) and arginine vasopressin (AVP). In chronic stress or chronic stimulation of the HPA axis, AVP assumes a larger role in the modulation of the HPA axis. ACTH stimulates the adrenal cortex to produce cortisol, a glucocorticoid. Low levels seem to heighten the perception of pain, which is a characteristic of people who have FS.

To assess the integrity of the HPA axis in people with FS, Crofford and colleagues (1994) measured urinary free cortisol over a 24-hour period and plasma cortisol in the morning and in the evening. The results showed significantly reduced cortisol in the urine of individuals with FS compared to the control group. In addition, the cortisol levels in the plasma of FS were significantly increased in the evening at the same time that the controls experienced a trough. This indicates a malfunction in the diurnal pattern of cortisol production in the group with FS. These researchers point out that these findings are consistent with those reported by McCain and Tilbe (1989). Neither the cause nor the effect of these findings in relation to FS is yet understood, according to these researchers.

Growth hormone (GH) is secreted by the pituitary gland and therefore is part of the HPA axis. In the early stage of a stress response, there is typically an elevated level of GH that drops to a subnormal level in prolonged stress (Chrousos and Gold 1992). If chronic pain is an example of prolonged stress, then this may be part of the explanation for low GH in people with FS as measured by Dr. Bennett and colleagues (1992). In this study, the researchers measured somatomedin-C (IGF-1, an insulin-like growth factor), which is a metabolite of GH, and found the blood level to be reduced in people with FS.

Another connection of the HPA axis to FS is its effect on the functions of cellular growth and repair. These two functions are apparently impaired in people with FS. Corresponding to this clinical feature is the fact that the level of DHEA (dehydroepiandrosterone), a steroid-type hormone responsible for cellular growth and development, is low in people with FS. How does DHEA fit into the HPA axis? First, the hypothalamus must stimulate the pituitary gland to elicit the production of growth hormone, cortisol, and DHEA. We have already noted that growth hormone is low in individuals with FS. From this point on, there seems to be a chain reaction of insufficient metabolites being formed at each point of breakdown. Normal amounts of GH are not available to stimulate the production of IGF-1. IGF-1 is a chemical that has the task of stimulating the adrenal glands to produce DHEA. As DHEA metabolizes, it forms DHEAS (dehydroepiandrosterone sulfate), which has been measured and found to be low in people with FS, rheumatoid arthritis, and osteoarthritis (Russell 1994a). Subjects with low levels of DHEAS also had low levels of serotonin and IGF-1. The researchers also found a correlation between a high perceived pain level of the subjects and low levels of DHEAS.

If DHEAS and IGF-1 levels are suppressed, then DHEA levels are probably also suppressed. Research regarding symptoms associated with aging, such as fatigue, forgetfulness, and muscle weakness, has shown that DHEA taken in small doses alleviated these symptoms. Dr. Samuel S. C. Yen conducted this research at the University of California at San Diego (*Daily Herald,* January 13, 1995). Perhaps low doses of DHEA could do the same for people with FS.

Dysfunction of the HPA axis may also be caused by substance P, an 11-amino acid peptide, which is a neurotransmitter for primary nociceptor afferents that make synaptic junctions with dendrites of neurons in the spinal cord dorsal horn (Piercey et al. 1981). Afferent neurons in the spinal cord normally release substance P in response to painful stimuli. However, if substance P is not modulated adequately, an individual's perception of pain will be heightened. Researchers discovered that the level of substance P in the cerebrospinal fluid (CSF) of people with FS is three times higher than normal (Vaerøy et al. 1988). This increased level of substance P suggests a major imbalance in the pain modulation system. These researchers also suggest that substance P can affect the sympathetic nervous system, especially in the event of Raynaud's or Raynaud's-like phenomena. A serendipitous finding of this study was that the FS patients who were also smokers had an even higher level of substance P in their CSF.

The next year, Vaerøy and colleagues published a follow-up study relating substance P and Raynaud's phenomenon (Vaerøy et al. 1989). Surprisingly, the researchers found that a cold pressor test resulted in significantly less vasoconstriction among the hands of people with FS even though they had indicated by prior survey that they did have Raynaud's. This study calls into question previous diagnoses of Raynaud's phenomenon. In this instance, there seemed to be hyporeactivity of the sympathetic nervous system. One possible explanation given was that this finding might indicate an "exhaustion of the system."

Substance P appears to be very active and very powerful in the symptomatology of people with FS and, therefore, deserves more comment. According to White and Helme (1985), substance P is found in the small-diameter nerve fibers in the skin. These fibers are sometimes found in association with small blood vessels. This fact may have some bearing on the extreme tenderness to touch that is experienced by some individuals with FS. The researchers also describe substance P as a vasodilator, which is probably the critical factor in initiating a neurogenic inflammatory response.

The other major component of the stress regulating system is the locus ceruleus-norepinephrine/autonomic (sympathetic) system, which is located in the brain stem (Chrousos and Gold 1992). To a large extent, this system dictates our "fight or flight" response. According to Dr. Leslie Crofford (1993), the series of responses for "fight or flight" can be elicited by three things: (1) psychological or emotional events, (2) metabolic and physiologic disturbances, and (3) inflammatory processes.

Fibromyalgia syndrome has been described as a condition in which the affected individual is in a constant state of "fight or flight" or at least has an overstimulated sympathetic nervous system. This state has also been termed *hypervigilance.* Dr. Robert Murphy (1990) of Ohio summed up this finding by saying that fibromyalgia patients "idle at 30 miles per hour." This concept is clearly supported by clinical observations of most people with FS who, by their own admission, are easily overstimulated. Perhaps this partially accounts for the typically stiff, tight muscles of people with FS. More importantly, this concept is supported by studies that indicate a reduced relaxation rate (Backman et al. 1988) and insufficient relaxation between contractions as observed with electromyography (Elert et al. 1992). This state-of-hypervigilance concept could also help explain the poor sleep architecture typical of the person with FS who awakes feeling unrefreshed and complains of being a light sleeper.

Perhaps the seemingly overstimulated sympathetic nervous system responses are caused by a hypersensitive sympathetic nervous system. They might also be caused by a minor imbalance between the sympathetic and parasympathetic nervous systems. For instance, the parasympathetic system could become less active than normal, leaving the sympathetic system overly powerful. In another scenario, both systems could become hyperactive or hypoactive. In the mitral valve prolapse syndrome literature, this imbalance is called *dysautonomia.* In *Confronting Mitral Valve Prolapse Syndrome,* Lyn Frederickson, M.S.N. (1988), suggests that "the pattern of dysautonomia may change over time, and the degree to which there is an imbalance may also change over time."

Sleep Disorder

What are some factors that could combine with the genetic predisposition to FS and lead to the manifestation of FS? One likely event is a sleep disorder. Sleep disorders are prevalent among people with FS and may contribute to the development of FS. This is not a new idea as Dr. Lue (1994) reports references from ancient cultures that related sleep and somatic complaints. In fact, several sleep disorders have been observed in people with FS. The sleep disorder most commonly seen in those who have FS is known as the alpha-delta sleep anomaly or the alpha intrusion anomaly. In this disturbed sleep pattern, the alpha waves that are characteristic of the light sleep stage invade the deep sleep stage and replace the delta waves. This anomaly seems to occur more in the first few hours of sleep than in the last few hours.

Many people with FS relate a nightly sleep pattern in which they feel they have just gotten to "good" sleep when it is time to arise in the morning. The individual awakens in the morning feeling unrested and "like a truck ran over me." In short, the person feels nonrestored; thus, this sleep disorder is also called *nonrestorative sleep.*

The bulk of the research on this aspect of FS has been conducted by Harvey Moldofsky, M.D., of Toronto. According to Dr. Moldofsky (1990), alpha waves have a frequency of 8 to 12 cycles per second and are noted on EEG during the drowsy stage of sleep. Stage 1 waves slow to 3 to 7 cycles per second. In stage 2, the waves speed up to 12 to 14 cycles per second and in deep, non-REM sleep the waves are very slow at 0.5 to 2 cycles per second. These very slow waves are called delta waves. In a large percentage of people with FS, alpha waves have replaced delta waves, depriving the patients of the deep restorative sleep that is so critical to good health (Moldofsky 1990).

In a well-known study (Moldofsky and Scarisbrick 1976), the deep sleep stage of healthy, sedentary subjects was disturbed by noise. This added disturbance led to FS-like symptoms, such as muscle pain, fatigue, and mood problems, in subjects under study. However, this deep sleep disruption did not induce pain in subjects who were aerobically fit. This finding indicates strongly that there is more than one important factor to consider in connecting the sleep anomaly to muscle pain.

Why is deep sleep referred to as restorative sleep? Apparently, the bodily repair of daily wear and tear occurs, or is at least set in motion, during the delta wave, or deep sleep, stage. One such important event is the repair of skeletal muscles. The process of repairing skeletal muscles also requires growth hormone (nutropin). This growth hormone is in short supply for people with FS, according to Robert Bennett, M.D. (Bennett et al. 1992). He measured the blood level of somatomedin-C (also called IGF-1) in 285 people with FS and 117 healthy individuals. Somatomedin-C is a breakdown product of growth hormone and is much easier to measure than the growth hormone itself. Levels of somatomedin-C were significantly lower among the group with FS. Another significant fact that Holl and colleagues (1991) found is that about 80% of a person's growth hormone is normally produced during stage 4 (deep) sleep. Since deep sleep is disrupted in people with FS and it appears that restorative functions are impaired, there appears to be a link between sleep and muscle pain.

Another contributing factor to decreased levels of growth hormone is lack of exercise. Separate studies by DeVries and colleagues (1991) and by Weltman and colleagues (1992) have shown an increase in growth hormone in healthy people following exercise. From these findings it might be concluded that people with FS could increase their levels of growth hormone if they exercised more. Another way of interpreting this finding is to look at it from the opposite view and wonder if the low levels of growth hormone in the individual with FS might make exercise more difficult. Consequently, the person with FS would develop more problems due to disuse of muscles and to decreased aerobic capacity.

Along that same line of thinking, Cuneo and colleagues (1991) found that administering growth hormone in the form of rhGH (recombinant DNA human GH) to adults with severe growth deficiency over a six-month period improved their VO2 max and their maximum power output. Their study suggests that positive gains are made in the type I muscle fibers rather than in the type II fibers.

Related to the growth hormone studies is the interesting research done by Jacobsen and colleagues (1990) in which they measured a protein that is closely linked to growth hormone production. In people with FS who have severe symptoms, the researchers found low levels of procollagen type III amino terminal peptide. Dr. Jacobsen suggests that the low levels of this procollagen peptide might be indicative of low collagen synthesis in people with FS. These low levels would pose a significant problem in view of the function of collagen, which is to provide the basis for development of connective tissue throughout the body. If this process is impaired, it might interfere with normal connective (muscle) repair. Apparently, this study investigated only people with FS who had severe symptoms. If further study reveals that this alteration in the procollagen peptide does not occur, or occurs to a lesser degree, in people with FS who have less severe symptoms, it might contribute to a better understanding of the wide range of severity of pain that is reported among people with FS.

Sleep is also considered necessary for modulating immunological responses. Some of the chemicals involved in the interaction between sleep and responses of the immunological system include interleukin-1 (IL-1), interleukin-2 (IL-2), muramyl dipeptide (a breakdown product of bacterial cell walls), vasoactive intestinal peptide, prostaglandin D-2, and factor S (Moldofsky et al. 1986, 1989). Studies in which immunological and endocrinological functions have been analyzed in relationship to sleep deprivation indicate that sleep deprivation causes significant alteration in the levels and functions of these substances. The converse appears to be true also—that alteration in these substances can produce a sleep disorder.

Dr. Moldofsky and colleagues (1986) found that normally the level of plasma IL-1 was at its peak at the onset of the delta stage of sleep. This was followed in half an hour by IL-2 reaching its peak level. While these two cytokines were at their peaks, the natural killer (NK) cell activity was very low. (Natural killer cells are a specific type of lymphocyte that select and kill certain tumor cells, micro-organisms, and cells infected by viruses [Mackinnon 1989]). To prove the existence of a connection between sleep and the immune system, Dr. Moldofsky and colleagues (1989) introduced sleep deprivation and then measured IL-1, IL-2, and NK cell activity again. As he predicted, significant changes were found. The levels of IL-1 and IL-2 were elevated and the NK cell activity was erratic. Of particular interest is the fact that elevated levels of IL-1 and IL-2 are known to cause muscle pain and fatigue.

Muramyl dipeptide is one of the chemicals involved in the interaction between sleep and immunological responses. When friendly bacteria are digested in the stomach, muramyl dipeptides are released from the bacterial walls and travel via the blood to activate serotonin receptors in the brain. These dipeptides become a link in normal serotonin function. Serotonin seems to be critical to normal, healthy sleep (Bennett 1993a). If a disruption occurs in the normal process of bacterial digestion, as would occur in the event of invasion by an infectious agent, then the serotonin function would likely be disrupted also (Krueger and Johannsen 1988).

Krueger and Johannsen (1988) also suggest that the balance of sleep-wake functions is achieved and maintained by complicated relationships between HPA axis hormones and several immunologically active peptides, which gives us an idea of the delicate balance and intricate nature of eventual successful treatment of FS.

In women, the hormonal cycle complicates the situation because the plasma IL-1 levels increase during the luteal phase in healthy women (Cannon and Dinarello 1985). Remember that Dr. Moldofsky and colleagues (1986) found that the plasma IL-1 level is normally at its peak at the onset of delta sleep. Perhaps the significance of Cannon and Dinarello's work in relation to FS is that some imbalance of the immunological system occurs because of the increase in IL-1 during the luteal phase.

Serotonin (5-Hydroxytryptamine)

A significant portion of the research on fibromyalgia has focused on the neurotransmitter serotonin, which is a metabolite of the essential amino acid tryptophan. We must obtain the supply of tryptophan we need from food sources because our bodies do not manufacture it. Serotonin is apparently involved in a number of functions that affect FS sufferers, such as sleep disorders and heightened pain perception. There is evidence that "serotoninergic pathways have been implicated in both the descending pathways inhibiting peripheral pain appreciation and in the complex pathways involved in the generation of sleep" (Bennett 1993a). Therefore, the fact that serotonin levels are low in some people with FS (Russell et al. 1987) is consistent with clinical findings that people with FS have increased perceptions of pain and disturbed sleep.

Several years ago, researchers determined that available tryptophan in the brain is low in people with FS (Yunus et al. 1992, Russell et al. 1989). This finding has spawned a great deal of new research. First, we will look at the metabolism of tryptophan, as discussed by I. Jon Russell, M.D., at the 1993 American College of Rheumatology meeting in San Antonio (Russell 1994b, 1994c). Usually, the metabolic breakdown of tryptophan produces serotonin, but sometimes a different pathway can occur due to overactivation by the enzyme IDO. In the alternate metabolic pathway, kynurenine (KYN) will be produced. If this happens too often, the level of serotonin will be reduced. A product of the KYN pathway is quinolic acid, which seems to cause anxiety and irritability. Incidentally, an increase in concentration of this acid is found in the brain as aging occurs.

Another very intriguing but small study indicates that female hormones may somehow cause the conversion of tryptophan to KYN in preference to serotonin. Further study about the metabolism of tryptophan may enlighten us about the prevalence of FS among women. Moldofsky (1994) looked at the female hormones in a sleep study in which he found that healthy women do not sleep as deeply during the second half of their cycle. He also found that there is less natural killer cell activity in women during that part of their cycle. A last note of interest from this discussion was that the KYN conversion route also occurs when the individual has consumed alcohol or received interferon therapy. (Interferon is used in chemotherapy and is also an infection fighter produced by the body.)

In a further investigation of the kynurenine pathway, Dr. Russell (1993a, 1993b) determined that the concentrations of several red blood cell nucleotides were reduced in people with FS, especially adenosine triphosphate (ATP), nicotinamide adenine dinucleotide phosphate (NADP), and nicotinamide adenine dinucleotide (NADH). However, there was no correlation between any of these levels and the perceived pain of people with FS.

With regard to the conversion of tryptophan to serotonin, there are several interesting findings. First, the serum level of serotonin, norepinephrine, and dopamine are all decreased in people with FS (Yunus et al. 1992). Dr. Russell and colleagues (Russell et al. 1992b) found that the levels of the metabolites of these three neurotransmitters are decreased in the spinal fluid as well. All three neurotransmitters (serotonin, norepinephrine, and dopamine) are considered to be important in directing the pituitary gland to order the production of growth hormone.

As mentioned previously, the sleep anomaly suppresses the production of growth hormone because of the decreased amount of time spent in the delta sleep stage. Research findings have indicated that there is likely a second factor at work in the suppression of growth hormone in people with FS—the decreased level of serotonin. Dr. Bennett's (Bennett et al. 1992) research on the concentration of somatomedin-C showed that growth hormone is low in people with FS. Dr. Russell's (1992) measurements of the serotonin metabolite 5-HIAA in the cerebrospinal fluid and Dr. Yunus's (1992) serum measurements indicated that serotonin levels are diminished in people with FS.

Another possible effect of decreased serotonin level is an increased perception of pain. There is some indication that serotonin is active in regulating the perception of pain via its inhibitory function in the hypothalamus. If there is not enough of the neurotransmitter present to modulate pain stimuli, then the pain perception would likely be elevated. This effect happens in combination with the fact that substance P, which heightens pain perception, is greatly increased in people with FS (Vaerøy et al. 1988). With these two abnormalities occurring simultaneously, the net effect is likely an elevated perception of pain.

The concentration of serotonin also affects the activity of natural killer cells. In the event of too little serotonin, the regulating monocytes fail to induce sufficient numbers of natural killer cells to become active. This explanation is consistent with the observation that the activity level of the natural killer cells is abnormally low in people with FS (Russell et al. 1988).

According to separate research by Peroutka (1990) and by Hamon and colleagues (1990), nine different serotonin receptor subtypes have been identified. These sites are very specific. In other words, a specific key is required to fit each lock. As a result, devising a pharmacological treatment becomes a much bigger challenge in that it is now obvious that one serotonin-enhancing drug will not be sufficient. Complicating the matter even further is the probability that each receptor site dysfunction affects pain modulation differently. It seems that some receptor sites affect anxiety, some affect depression, and some affect anger and panic. It is not yet known how to determine which receptor subtype is at fault in an individual, nor how to prescribe medication accordingly.

Nutrition

Travell and Simons (1983) attribute some of the problems associated with myofascial pain syndromes to nutritional inadequacies. In their book on myofascial pain they offer details on the roles played by various vitamins and minerals and suggest the probable effects each nutrient might have on muscle and nerve function. They found that vitamin therapy was necessary in treating myofascial pain in about 50% of their patients. They state that "vitamin inadequacy apparently increases the irritability of myofascial trigger points by several mechanisms: impairment of the energy metabolism needed for the contraction of muscles and increased irritability of the nervous system" (Travell and Simons 1992). Until recently, there has been a paucity of reported research in this area. Now the interest in the nutritional aspects of fibromyalgia is growing.

Recently, there have been some reports of empirical findings on the effects of the augmentation of magnesium in the diet. People with FS took extra magnesium and reported that they felt better. Perhaps it was this type of report that led researchers to look further. The new interest in magnesium may also have stemmed from a 1986 study on the high-energy compounds showing that ATP is low in people with FS and that ATP synthesis depends on an enzyme and magnesium (Bengtsson, Henriksson, and Larsson 1986a). Dr. Goldberg (1992) indicates that magnesium is important in reactions that involve ATP and that a deficiency is associated with metabolic and neurologic dysfunction.

Daniel Clauw, M.D. (1994b), suspected that people with FS were deficient in magnesium. To determine whether this was true, he used magnetic resonance spectroscopy (MRS) to ascertain the level of magnesium in the gastrocnemius muscle of 20 people with FS. He found that the lower the level of magnesium, the higher the person's level of pain.

In another experiment, he loaded his research subjects with magnesium (Clauw 1994a). He reasoned that people who were deficient in magnesium would retain more of the magnesium than those who had an adequate level. The results showed that the magnesium retention rate for normal subjects was 40% whereas the rate was 70% for people with FS, which confirmed Dr. Clauw's suspicion.

In another study, Thomas Romano, M.D. (1994), found lower red blood cell magnesium levels in 100 people with FS in comparison to a healthy control group. However, the plasma levels of magnesium were within normal limits for the people with FS.

Abraham and Flechas (1992) hypothesized that FS results from a deficiency of substances needed for adenosine triphosphate (ATP) synthesis. They point out the many junctures at which malic acid and magnesium are necessary in the process of making ATP. In their study, they administered 300 to 600 milligrams of magnesium per day and 1200 to 2400 milligrams of malic acid per day to 15 people with FS. This regime led to reduced pain within 48 hours. Statistically significant improvement of pain at trigger point sites was seen at 4 and 8 weeks. Return of pain occurred within 48 hours of switching to a placebo.

According to Lyn Frederickson (1988), magnesium is decreased due to stress. Also, she advises against drinking soft drinks because they contain such high levels of phosphates, which "leach magnesium from the body."

Travell and Simons (1992) also cite magnesium deficiency as a causative factor in poor absorption of thiamine (vitamin B1), which is critical in energy metabolism within the Krebs cycle. Dr. C. Norman Shealy (1987) has observed clinically that pyroxidine (vitamin B6) was low in 150 people with chronic pain. His study did not focus on individuals with FS but on people with chronic pain. Pertaining to fibromyalgia, he notes that vitamin B6 must be present for the conversion of tryptophan to 5-hydroxytryptamine (serotonin). He also notes that B6 is less available in today's typically highly refined diet than it used to be. Abraham and Flechas (1992) point out that the activation of B6 requires a magnesium-dependent phosphate transfer reaction. Therefore, it seems that magnesium must be available for the conversion of tryptophan to serotonin.

Dr. Shealy (1987) also points out the impact of smoking on the blood level of vitamin B6. Eighty percent of the smokers in his study were deficient in vitamin B6 and only 35 percent of the nonsmokers were deficient.

Travell and Simons (1992) note that vitamin B6 deficiency affects other nutrients and processes. For example, reduced B6 leads to increased excretion of vitamin C and poor synthesis of niacin (nicotinic acid). They explain that B6 is vital in the breakdown of tryptophan as it metabolizes to niacin. Of special interest for people with FS is the fact that vitamin B6 helps with neurotransmitter synthesis and metabolism, which includes serotonin. Another important substance that is often in short supply in people with FS is growth hormone. Vitamin B6 is important in its production.

Eisinger, Plantamurs, and Ayavou (1994) set out to determine whether an impairment of carbohydrate metabolism might be a contributing or causal factor in FS. They learned that people with FS exhibited a decrease in ATP, an increase in pyruvate by 84%, and a diminished serum lactate maximal increase. An increase in the pyruvate to lactate ratio was also noted. This abnormality has also been associated with thiamine (vitamin B1) deficiency. Another abnormal finding concerned the deficit of muscular lactase dehydrogenase (LDH) iso-enzymes, which is also reported in muscular dystrophy (Ibrahim, Essam, and Kottke 1974). It is suggested that glycolysis could be impaired by GH abnormalities. Such impairment can lead to poor activation of thiamine and to decreased levels of serotonin. According to biochemist Dr. Stephen Goldberg (1992), vitamin B1 deficiency can lead to general weakness and pins-and-needles sensations.

Vitamin C might be helpful to people with FS if poor collagen synthesis is proved to be a factor in the condition, as is suggested by Jacobsen and colleagues (1990). They found low levels of procollagen type III amino terminal peptide in people with FS who had severe symptoms. They concluded that these low levels would diminish collagen synthesis, which would affect all connective tissues in the body. According to Leadbetter (1992), ascorbic acid (vitamin C) is required for collagen production. This relationship has been further elucidated by Dr. Goldberg (1992), who explains that vitamin C is essential for the hydroxylation of proline, which yields hydroxyproline, one of the chief components of collagen. Vitamin C may also be important in the production of corticosteroids and epinephrine (Goldberg 1992). These substances are being measured by FS researchers.

Dr. Goldberg (1992) also mentions that corn is low in tryptophan. People who eat a lot of corn may experience a niacin deficiency, since niacin is a product of one of the breakdown pathways of tryptophan. Niacin (nicotinic acid) is part of the NADH molecule (nicotinamide adenine dinucleotide), which is important in certain red blood cell nucleotides (Russell 1993b) and in the Krebs cycle (Goldberg 1992). A deficiency could decrease a person's energy and ability to do work.

Some evidence indicates that carbohydrates are generally high in tryptophan and that loading with carbohydrates after fasting may increase brain serotonin (Leathwood 1987). However, this result has been witnessed only in rats thus far. The author suggests that the rate of tryptophan transport across the blood-brain barrier is improved by this dietary modification.

> *The mechanism by which diet (or tryptophan [TRP]) is thought to influence 5HT [brain serotonin] synthesis involves the following sequence: the composition of food consumed changes plasma levels of the large neutral amino acids (LNAA), which affect, in turn, the rate of TRP transport into the brain, brain TRP levels and hence the rate of 5HT (5-hydroxytryptonine) synthesis. It has been suggested that, by this mechanism, dietary interventions might influence a range of behaviors and brain functions linked to serotonergic neurotransmission* (Leathwood 1987, 143).

Finally, alcohol plays a role in the metabolism of tryptophan (Russell 1993b). The ingestion of alcohol biases the conversion of tryptophan to follow the kynurenine (KYN) pathway, which leads to the formation of quinolic acid. Apparently, this chemical is found in the aging brain and seems to cause anxiety and irritability. The critical factor for the person with FS is that if tryptophan is being converted along the KYN pathway, then it is not producing serotonin. Because serotonin has been shown to be important in the FS process, people need to do what they can in order to boost serotonin in their bodies.

Psychological Factors

Psychological distress or disease has long been blamed for the symptoms associated with FS. One reason underlying this belief is the lack of solid, objective findings for diagnosing the disease, such as a laboratory test would provide. Perhaps now the tender point site assessment will qualify as sound physical evidence. Another reason for assuming a psychological basis is the fact that people with FS often appear to be depressed and complain of symptoms that are commonly associated with depression, such as tiredness, difficulty sleeping, anxiety, irritable bowels, and headaches.

Research has shown that the majority of people with FS do not exhibit psychological illness as the cause of their symptoms. Dr. Goldenberg (1986) used the National Institute of Mental Health's Diagnostic Interview Schedule to determine whether individuals with FS also had a psychological illness. He found that only 21% of people with FS had a psychiatric diagnosis concurrently with FS. Interestingly, 57% of the group had a past history of some psychiatric illness, usually depression. He also found that first-degree relatives of people with FS suffered from major depression more commonly than first-degree relatives of people with rheumatoid arthritis. Some studies indicate that a high percentage of people with FS experience depression but it appears that depression would occur as a result of having a chronic pain syndrome. High medical bills surely contribute to the anxieties and fears of people with FS as many of them have searched for years for relief from pain, seen many doctors, and tried numerous medications. Some have even undergone surgery.

Another fact that might implicate psychiatric illness as an etiological explanation of FS is that similar medications are used to treat FS and depression. The tricyclic family of drugs has been used effectively for both conditions, although the dosage used for people with FS is much less than that used to treat depression. In fact, at the lower dosages it is inappropriate to refer to the tricyclics as antidepressants. The purpose of the tricyclic drug is to boost the serotonin level. Lower dosages are usually sufficient for people with FS. Another reason it has been assumed that psychological problems are the cause, rather than the result, of FS is that stress often exacerbates patients' symptoms.

Dr. I. Jon Russell (1992) has stated that "The incidence of depression in FS is the same as it is in rheumatoid arthritis and no one says that depression causes RA." There is some indication that 70% of people with FS have had major depression at some time during their lives. Ahles and colleagues (1984) found that figure to be consistent with the lifetime depression percentage for people with rheumatoid arthritis and for a control group.

In a review of studies about psychological factors in people with FS, Dr. Yunus (1994) concludes that FS is not generated by psychological distress. He points out that most studies regarding depression and FS have shown that people with FS are no more depressed than the control group. This finding was established when people with FS were compared to people with rheumatoid arthritis on the Zung Depression Inventory (Ahles, Yunus, and Masi 1987). When compared to a control group from a primary care clinic using the Beck Depression Inventory, people with FS did not exhibit greater depression (Clark et al. 1985).

Global anxiety is another characteristic of people with FS, which Dr. Yunus (1994) found in 60% of FS patients through the use of a questionnaire. This symptom probably corresponds to the effect of stress on FS. Dr. Yunus and colleagues (1991) found that stress, depression, and anxiety can be used to predict the severity of pain in people with FS.

Chemical differences between people with FS and people with depression have also been shown. For instance, 3H-imipramine binding is different in the two conditions (Kravitz et al. 1992). Another chemical difference was noted in the cortisol levels of individuals with FS compared to individuals with depression. Crofford (1993) found that the cortisol level is reduced in the FS population. Dr. M. Yunus (1993) made the comparison of people with FS and people with depression by saying, "Earlier the question was raised about whether depression and FS are similar syndromes, overlapping syndromes, et cetera. It looks to me that, biologically, they are different conditions. In depression you have hypercortisolism, whereas in FS patients, you have hypocortisolism."

Yunus and colleagues (1991) point out that even though pain perception is affected by psychological distress, the tender points, sleep disturbance, subjective swelling, and paresthesia "do not correlate with the psychological profiles of fibromyalgia patients."

Measuring instruments for mental stress, such as the Hassles Scale and the Life Events Inventory, have been applied to people with FS. They rate higher for mental stress than people with rheumatoid arthritis and normal controls on daily hassles on the Hassles Scale (Dailey et al. 1990) and on the Life Events Inventory (Ahles et al. 1984). However, in the Dailey study the people with FS scored lower on major life stresses.

In Germany, a controlled study involving 65 people with FS and 53 people with rheumatoid arthritis pointed to more childhood trauma and, therefore, increased risk factors for psychological distress, among the people with FS (Schuessler and Konermann 1993). People with FS also perceived their pain as greater and were more elaborate in describing their pain than the people with arthritis. Still, the researchers concluded that FS is not a psychogenic disease.

The reference to childhood trauma hints at a topic that has received some attention as a cause of FS, which is that many people with FS give a history of being the target of physical or sexual abuse. Two recent studies found a slightly higher percentage of FS patients than controls who reported a history of being abused, substance abuse, or eating disorders (Boisset-Pioro 1995 and Taylor 1995). However, it is important to note that the incidence was not statistically significant. Both sets of researchers noted a statistical association between the occurrence of FS and the number of associated symptoms with the reported frequency of abuse. In an editorial in the same journal, Hudson and Pope (1995) warn of the pitfalls of such retrospective studies in which heavy reliance is made on victims' memories. They point out that erroneous causal relationships might be deduced. For instance, the association between childhood sexual abuse and FS could possibly be less direct than is readily apparent. Genetics or substance abuse might actually be the link. They also say that people who are abusing a substance are more likely to abuse a family member physically or sexually. Also, the tendency to substance abuse has a genetic factor.

On the other hand, Wolfe (1993b, 2) says that "by any measure fibromyalgia patients have higher depression scores than all of the other disease groups." This assessment does not indicate whether the depression was present prior to the onset of FS or whether the stress of the condition might have caused the depression. Wolfe acknowledges that not all individuals with FS have depression.

There is also some indication that depression may be associated with low levels of growth hormone. People with FS are also known to have low levels of growth hormone (Bennett et al. 1992). Growth hormone, Bennett and colleagues found, "not only acts to make the body physically stronger and spryer, it also alters the chemistry of the brain. One of the changes they found is an increase in beta endorphin, a 'good feeling' brain chemical that is linked to memory impairment and depression when it is low" (Kotulak 1994, 3). This comment seems to suggest that bringing growth hormone levels to normal could help improve memory loss and depression, two conditions often associated with FS.

There is a generally accepted rumor that people with FS share a specific personality type—that they are compulsive and perfectionistic. Dr. Goldenberg (1986) suggests that this rumor was derived from results of testing with the Minnesota Multiphasic Personality Inventory (MMPI) and other psychological evaluations that were inappropriately applied to people with FS. These instruments have not been validated for diagnostic use in questions of personality disorders. He reports that in some situations the testing was applied only to people with such severe problems that they were hospitalized. Other studies have suffered from similar referral biases. He reminds us that biologic and behavioral changes occur with any chronic condition. In recognition of such changes, he conducted a controlled study utilizing cognitive behavior treatment, stress reduction, and meditation. Goldenberg and colleagues (1994) found a 67% improvement of the symptoms of FS among 78 people studied. This 10-week program involved some individuals with FS who had found minimal help with tricyclic and analgesic medications, education, and exercise. Some participants improved by more than 50% and a few experienced nearly complete abatement of symptoms. Psychological distress decreased by 33% in the subjects studied.

Medications

The literature abounds with pharmacological studies in relationship to FS. Indeed, new medications are being introduced in rapid succession. Each one supposedly has fewer side effects than its parent drug. The most often mentioned medication seems to be the tricyclic family, especially amitriptyline (elavil) and cyclobenzaprine (flexeril). Amitriptyline is most effective for FS in low dosages and is believed to help by boosting the available serotonin in the body. Dr. Goldenberg (1989) noted significant benefit with its usage, but this was short-lived in the majority of the subjects. In a double-blind crossover study, researchers confirmed Dr. Goldenberg's finding of significant improvement in the pain level with the use of low dosages of amitriptyline (Scudds et al. 1989).

In a study comparing amitriptyline and naproxen, Dr. Goldenberg found 10 to 50 milligrams of amitriptyline to be more beneficial than 1000 milligrams of naproxen (Goldenberg, Felson, and Dinerman 1986). Other nonsteroidal anti-inflammatory drugs (NSAIDs) used alone have proven to be ineffective also (Goldenberg, Felson, and Dinerman 1986; Yunus, Masi, and Aldag 1989). Dr. Goldenberg's study did show that the combination of amitriptyline and naproxen was slightly more helpful than amitriptyline alone.

A triazolobenzodiazepine called alprazolam (xanax) and ibuprofen (NSAID) have been studied in two separate, controlled trials. In one study of 78 patients, the combination was more effective than a placebo or either drug alone (Russell et al. 1991). In another study by Kravitz and colleagues (1994), each drug administered alone was more efficacious than the placebo or the combination of the two. Many possible reasons for the dissimilar outcomes of the two studies were discussed. Nonetheless, the results were inconclusive and confusing.

Another tricyclic that has been the subject of large trials is cyclobenzaprine. Even though most patients taking tricyclics perceive that they are sleeping better, Reynolds and colleagues (1991) did not see an improvement in the alpha intrusion disturbance in people taking cyclobenzaprine. Neither was there improvement in pain, tender points, or mood. But there was a decrease in evening fatigue and an increase in total sleep time.

In a 12-week study, cyclobenzaprine (flexeril) was more effective than the placebo in reducing fatigue and pain and in improving sleep (Bennett et al. 1988). The effectiveness of this drug was supported by another study in 1989, although that study was "unblinded" by subjects who identified the drug (Quimby et al. 1989).

The use of corticosteroids for FS is worthless, according to a double-blind study in which 15 milligrams per day of prednisone was only as effective as the placebo (Clark, Tindall, and Bennett 1985).

A nonbenzodiazepine hypnotic called zopiclone was studied in a double-blind test over 8 weeks. Nearly all subjects who took the zopiclone experienced marked improvement in their sleep and in their pain and morning stiffness (Gronblad et al.

1993). The abnormal alpha delta sleep pattern was confirmed in people with FS and treated with mianserin with positive results (Herisson et al. 1989). Patients took 10-30 mg of mianserin each evening and the majority of subjects noted a decrease in widespread pain and an improvement in sleep. This was a small study but, based on the findings, the researchers suggest the use of sedative antidepressant drugs.

After discussion of the various medications at the National Seminar on Fibrositis/Fibromyalgia in April, 1990, Dr. George Waylonis, a researcher who has FS, offered that he often took only an antihistamine at night to help reduce his sleep disturbance (Waylonis 1990).

Dr. Goldenberg (1994b) has summarized that although some medications have been proven to help some individuals with FS, no one medication has yet been found to be effective in a majority of cases. He is most hopeful that "if specific neurohormonal deficiencies can be identified, a specific treatment approach could be developed. However, it is unlikely that a single medication or simple therapeutic approach will be highly effective in a complicated, chronic pain disorder, such as fibromyalgia, and investigators, as well as patients, must be open to trying a number of different therapeutic modalities" (Goldenberg 1994b).

Capsaicin is an example of a different therapeutic modality. Capsaicin is an ointment sold under the brand names Zostrix and Capzasin P. The main ingredient is capsaicin, which comes from Hungarian red peppers. Usually it causes intense burning when applied to the skin. Supposedly it stimulates the release of substance P and causes the depletion of substance P from the skin (White and Helme 1985). Some people with FS have found that it relieves the pain of trigger points. These results are anecdotal thus far.

Physical Therapy Management

As a physical therapist, treating individuals with FS provides a mixture of excitement and challenge, as well as frustration. There is excitement in realizing you are part of the early stages of understanding this condition. There is challenge in that it requires going beyond yourself and your training in order to become a partner with the client and discover the best program for each individual. There is no definite protocol because clients present with a broad variety of symptoms, precipitating factors, and functional levels. You will need to use your knowledge in creative ways, to use your empathy, and to be patient with very small steps forward. Finally, there is frustration in wanting to help more but being hindered by the current understanding of the condition, which is quite limited.

Since no one yet knows the source of problems in FS, we are faced with treating the peripheral symptoms rather than the source. There is also frustration in seeing such slow progress. Unfortunately, the therapist's frustration can lead to the delivery of poor treatment. It has been said that the sufferer who does not get well meets primitive human behavior called *treatment*. Let us be sure that the same cannot be said about our approach. Remember that "Pain is a symptom which has been difficult to confirm and to quantify but that does not excuse the medical community from developing new methods for doing so. Most of the pain experienced by patients has physiological or biochemical explanation. It is not the patient's responsibility to change her disease into something we know more about. Rather, it is our task to better understand the problem she has" (Russell 1993a, 3-4).

As a therapist treating clients with FS, you must accept that you will not see the dramatic or complete results that give so much satisfaction. Keep in mind that your task is to alleviate pain and help increase the client's functional level. These goals are not so different from the goals we have for other clients. The difference is that we know at the outset the pain alleviation will probably be temporary and that the precipitating factors can be many. You must help ferret out the probable precipitating factors and teach the client whatever methods you have in your repertoire that can minimize the effects of those precipitating factors.

Examples of common precipitating factors are:

- poorly designed work sites
- posture
- trauma
- emotional or physical stress
- poor sleep quality
- environmental sensitivities
- diet
- weather
- lack of exercise
- too much exercise

When trying to alleviate the pain and discomfort of FS, a helpful analogy is the peeling of an onion. Each layer represents a portion of the pain. With each layer that is removed, some portion of the pain is minimized. If several layers can be eliminated, then the client is going to feel much better, although perhaps not completely free of pain. If improvement is even 50%, then the client is going to be much more functional and the quality of life is going to be much better. Some of the tools that you, as a therapist, can use to peel back the various layers of the FS pain are:

- postural correction
- ergonomic instruction
- relaxation techniques
- aerobic work
- soft tissue work
- gentle strengthening
- modalities
- sleep position
- stretching
- education
- reassurance
- patience

"Of critical importance is the ability to convey the importance of fibromyalgia and chronic fatigue syndrome as possible diagnoses, their legitimacy as diagnoses with potential severity and disability, and the caring rather than curing nature of therapy" (Schwenk 1992). In other words, at least one layer of the client's pain is removed by having the FS diagnosis validated by you. You will not be able to cure these clients, so your level of caring will be even more important than with most clients.

History Taking

Recording the client's history is of prime importance in any evaluation that a therapist performs. When designing a therapeutic program and setting goals for a client, it is always helpful to know the details of mode of onset, pattern of symptoms, and the status of the patient prior to the incident. In dealing with FS, the history-taking process assumes even greater importance because the accepted body of knowledge about FS is incomplete at this time. Therefore, we need all the clues we can gather in order to design an effective treatment program for the individual client.

Another dimension of therapy that is often unappreciated by therapists is the client's simple need to tell his or her story. In most cases, no other health professional that the person with FS has seen has allowed the opportunity for relating the entire saga. This can be a stressor for the client for several reasons. One reason is that the client knows all the facts have not been gathered by anyone and senses that the basis for understanding the condition lies in a complete history. Of course, it can be very time consuming for a therapist to listen to the client's story and may cause stress for the busy therapist. However, the time spent is well worthwhile for a couple of reasons: the patient will reveal much that will help you determine how to facilitate progress, trust will be established, and some of the client's anxiety will be relieved. Taking time to listen is especially critical when working with clients who have FS because they are often bewildered and uneasy about the diagnosis as well as other people's reactions to it.

By listening carefully, you can learn about the client's lifestyle, recurring life events, stressors and triggers, level of function, and recreation interests. Sometimes you will find that the client has another medical problem that has been lumped in with the FS diagnosis but which needs to be approached separately. Or you may realize that the person is suffering from a sleep disturbance that has not been addressed by the physician. This is important because clients with FS do not seem to make progress without some improvement in their sleep.

Sleep disorders are very common in people with FS, especially the alpha intrusion disorder (see pages 35 to 38 for a more complete discussion of this sleep disorder). Restless leg syndrome and insomnia are also reported by those with FS. Clients are usually aware if they have restless legs or insomnia but often do not realize they have the alpha intrusion disorder. It is characterized on EEG by alpha waves intruding into the delta (non-REM) stage of sleep, thus reducing the amount of time the person spends in deep sleep. The clinical manifestation is feeling "like a truck ran over me" upon waking in the morning. For this reason, it is also known as nonrestorative sleep. If you ask a client about sleep problems, the client may not even be aware of any. But if you ask the client how he or she feels upon waking in the morning, the client will typically report feeling exhausted, run over, beaten up, or sore. Consistent with good history taking, you must ask questions correctly so that you are not misled by the response.

If the patient does reveal an apparent sleep disorder, then the problem needs to be addressed pharmacologically by a physician. Currently, the treatment of choice is serotonin-boosting medication, which facilitates the deep sleep stage. Good sleep hygiene practices also help to some degree and should be encouraged. They include eliminating alcohol and caffeine from the diet, exercising regularly, utilizing a relaxation technique, and instituting a regular bedtime. Other anecdotal aids to better sleep are drinking a glass of milk at bedtime (for the tryptophan) and having a constant sound in the bedroom, such as a fan or a sound machine. Wearing warm bedclothes and socks also helps. Some people have reported improvement in sleep after eating protein at bedtime.

Asking the right questions is also important for finding out about any cognitive dysfunction that the client may be having and attributing to other causes. Ask the patient about any memory problems, trouble with problem solving, and difficulty with word retrieval. While the exact nature of cognitive dysfunction associated with FS has not been delineated yet, letting the client know that it is often part of FS may be helpful. Such a discussion might lead you to uncover other symptoms such as global anxiety and concern that "I've turned into a crabby person." This type of comment may be an opener for a conversation about coping with a chronic problem and the effect of the situation on relationships. This is an ideal juncture for you to suggest that the client add another facet to the treatment regime: counseling. Recommend psychologists in your area who are well versed in fibromyalgia.

Physical Evaluation

The typical starting point for a new client in physical therapy is an evaluation. A complete evaluation provides a guide for designing a treatment plan. Your evaluation is rarely finished at the first visit as you will be continually re-evaluating the client. A reproducible evaluation form for recording your client evaluation is included on pages 57 to 58 for your use. A discussion of some of the important components of your evaluation follows.

1. ***Measurement of the range of motion (ROM) of the joints in the affected area.***

   If a person complains of pain and stiffness in the upper back and neck area, you will naturally assess the cervical ROM and the scapular rhythm. You will probably measure the shoulder ROM also. If there are problems in the lower back, you will assess trunk and hip range and flexibility. This is a usual procedure in any evaluation. However, in this case note carefully what the client says because in performing the requested range of motion the client with FS will often experience a greater increase in pain in the side toward which the movement is occurring. For example, the client will experience greater pain in the left upper trapezius with left side-bending of the neck than in the right upper trapezius. There may be the discomfort of stretching in the right upper trapezius, but the pain felt in the left upper trapezius will be of a different quality. Sometimes the pain may be described as a burning or aching. The client may say, "It makes me feel weak," or that it leads to radiating pain. Typically, passive range of motion is not limited, but quite often the pain limits the active range of motion and the patient may say, "I just can't do it."

2. ***Assessment of muscle strength and flexibility.***

   Keep in mind that pain alone may be the limiting factor, so it is not necessary to do a specific and detailed manual muscle test. In fact, such a process would likely precipitate a flare-up of symptoms if the client is able to tolerate it at all. A gross assessment of the client's state of general conditioning is usually sufficient. Clients with FS are typically deconditioned, although you will likely encounter some who are "overconditioned," such as clients who are aerobic dance instructors.

   Flexibility may be impeded by spasm, trigger points, or actual muscle shortening. Any muscle can be involved, but some of the most common ones to check for length are the levator scapulae muscles, upper trapezius muscles, pectoralis minor and major muscles, paravertebral muscles, trunk rotators, hamstrings, and gastrocnemius muscles. These tightnesses are sometimes secondary to inactivity rather than due to FS.

3. *Soft tissue assessment by palpation.*

In order to make this assessment, you need to have some knowledge of how normal tissue feels. You also need to know which muscle is superficial and which muscle lies deeper. Then you palpate and identify what you feel and observe, such as spasm, twitch response, taut bands, ropy areas, or knots. Map as much information as you can on a body chart.

When you begin to palpate, you must use very light pressure until you have determined whether the client can tolerate it. If the client tolerates the light pressure, then gradually increase your pressure and sink deeper into the muscle tissues. You need to keep communication open as you do this, constantly asking for the client's response to your pressure. For your records, you might want to use the severity scale proposed by Dr. I. Jon Russell and colleagues (1986).

They suggest that you use 4 kilograms of pressure (enough to cause blanching of the fingernail bed) as your standard. If there is no tenderness at a site, give a "0." If there is tenderness but no physical response, use a "1." If there is tenderness and some physical response, such as wincing or moving away, assign a "2." If there is a "jump sign" or the patient sharply withdraws, give a "3." If the client cannot allow the examiner to touch the site at all, use a "4." A tender point index is obtained by adding up the scores for all 18 sites. This index can be ascertained again at a later time to check progress. This detailed evaluation method may be more useful in research than in a busy clinic setting. A variation of this method might be more useful; for instance, grading only the tender points that are bothersome and mapping them well. Some of the points you will need to treat may not be among the ACR's 18 sites (see pages 10-11).

Examine the soft tissue bilaterally regardless of the client's complaints. In other words, if the client complains of pain in the right shoulder area and the right lower back area but never on the left side, you should still examine the tissue on the left side as well as the right side. Remember that one of the defining characteristics of FS is that it is a bilateral condition. If you fail to evaluate bilaterally then you surely will not treat bilaterally. If you treat only the right side, for instance, eventually the client will say that the pain has really subsided on the right side but has "moved" to the left side. You could have saved some time by checking both sides initially. An explanation for this occurrence is probably that the left-sided latent trigger points eventually become active. Another explanation might be that by reducing the stimulus of the right-sided pain, the client then realizes the discomfort on the left side. Sometimes the pain does "move" in that different tender points react at different times in response to a variety of precipitating factors.

Usually your palpatory sense will correlate with comments from the patient such as, "You're on one!" or "That's really tender." Some clients may be alarmed to find that your pressure on one site causes radiating symptoms, such as numbness, tingling, or pain. Sometimes clients are so tender they are unable to tolerate this exploration until a later session. These are the clients who might tell you they have difficulty bearing the weight of their clothes.

You will find that it is necessary in some cases to assess the soft tissue in different positions in order to get a complete picture of an area. For example, it seems that the upper trapezius and levator are more readily assessed in the seated position, but it is much easier to assess the thoracic aspect of the scapular musculature if the patient is sidelying or prone (see figure 1).

4. *Posture assessment: sitting and standing.*

Be sure to check the client's posture in the seated and in the standing positions. Then ask the client what position is assumed for the majority of each day. Perhaps the client works at a desk, or on an assembly line, or drives a truck. Assess the patient in the work position.

Because the discomfort caused by postural imbalances often compounds the muscular pain of FS, correcting a person's posture will usually offer some measure of relief and eliminate a precipitating factor. Sometimes the postural deviation is minimal. Even so, this can be a factor that needs to be addressed. Often you will see a forward head and rounded shoulders posture with an unstable lumbar area. Also, you will frequently find poor scapular rhythm and stabilization in these clients (see figure 2).

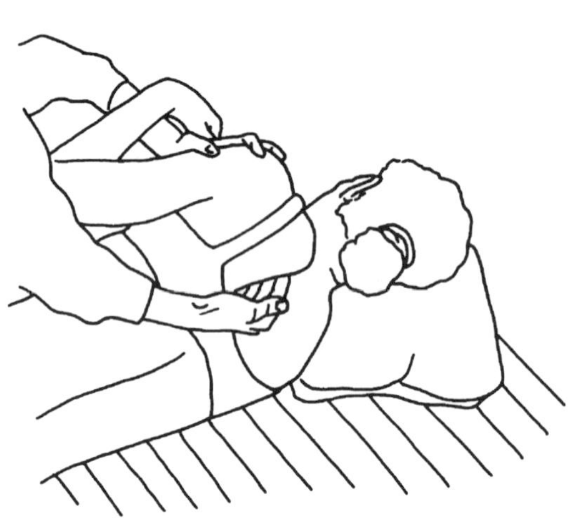

Figure 1. **Method for Assessing and Treating Tissue between Scapula and Thorax**

Note that the therapist's left arm and hand support the patient's left arm in slight external rotation while the therapist uses the left hand to push the shoulder posteriorly. This method gives some slack to the middle trapezius and rhomboids so that the fingers of the therapist's right hand can palpate along the thoracic aspect of the vertebral border of the scapula. Often there will be tender/trigger points there. This is one area that is impossible for the patient to work on independently.

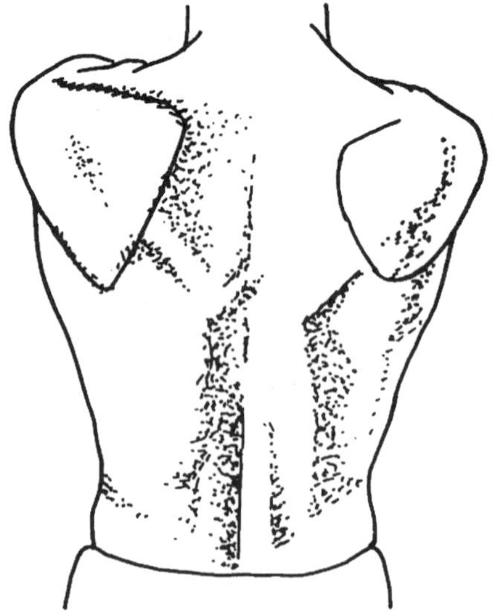

Figure 2. **Asymmetry of Scapulae**

Assess the symmetry of the scapulae in static position and during elevation of the shoulders. Note any asymmetry, as seen in the figure. Determine what is causing the asymmetry and treat accordingly. In this figure, note the excessively abducted inferior angle of the right scapula and depressed level of the superior angle. This probably represents relative weakness in the mid and lower trapezius.

5. ***Work site assessment.***

Ask the client about daily activities. Get a clear idea of the physical demands of these activities and whether they are repetitive or static in nature. Assume the postures yourself to get a sense of what the client's body must do. For instance, if the patient is a violinist, ask for a demonstration of the playing position. Then try it yourself and assess the stresses. If the client works at a computer, ask about desk height, chair height, position of the monitor, position of the keyboard, the lighting, chair style, and the position of the air conditioning vent. For how long does the client remain in one position? Even if the posture is perfect, remaining static will increase the discomfort. Show the client ways to change and alleviate the static positioning, such as scapular retractions or shoulder rolls. Finally, remember to ask the client if there is anything specific about the job that aggravates the symptoms.

6. ***Special tests.***

To assure yourself and the patient that anything and everything that is bothersome is not being attributed to FS without proper evaluation, you must perform any special tests that you feel will help determine whether a symptom is signaling another pathology. A few examples of special tests are Spurling's test for neck and radiating pain, apprehension and impingement signs when shoulder pain is present, and straight leg raising test when low back pain is a complaint.

Fibromyalgia Evaluation

Date: _________________________ Name: ____

Age: __________ Medications: ____

Physician: ____

Sport/Occupation: ____

Subjective Evaluation

History

How long have you been symptomatic? ____

Was the onset or exacerbation related to physical or emotional trauma, viral illness, birth of a baby, surgery, or nothing in particular? (provide detailed description) _______________________________

____

____

Other medical conditions or surgeries? (specifically, irritable bowel syndrome, mitral valve prolapse, Raynaud's phenomenon, or chronic fatigue syndrome) ________________________________

Symptoms

Energy Level: ____

Sleep Dysfunction: How do you feel upon awakening in the morning? Are you rested? ____________________

   Insomnia? _________ Restless legs? _________ Interrupted by pain? _________

Cognitive Dysfunction (memory, problem solving, other): ________________________________

Paresthesia: ____

(*Therapists:* please remember that the pattern of many paresthesias and referred pain is not consistent with dermatomal patterns. Be sure to consult the works of Travell and Simon regarding pain patterns associated with tender/trigger points.)

Pain: aching _____ burning _____ sharp _____

   throbbing _____ constant _____ intermittent _____

   other ____

Pain Perception (rate 0 to 10)

   Now: _____ Worst: _____ Best: _____

Pattern of Pain

Precipitating factors: Weather? _____ Stress? _____

   Environmental sensitivities? _____

   Other? ____

Nutrition concerns: Caffeine? _____ Alcohol? _____

   Smoking? _____ Water intake? _____

   Vitamin/mineral supplements? _____

Work site/recreational needs: _________________________

____

Sites of pain and paraesthesiae

0 = *hyposensitive*
II = *hypersensitive*
2 = *pain*
+ = *tenderness*

Fibromyalgia Evaluation (continued)

Objective Evaluation

Range of Motion: ____

Flexibility Tests: ____

Resisted Tests: ____

Posture: Forward head _______   Rounded shoulders _______   Kyphosis _______

Flattened lordosis (cervical, lumbar) _______   Abducted scapulae (static and dynamic assessment) _______

Winging scapulae (static and dynamic assessment) _______   Scoliosis _______   Hypermobility of joints _______

Pronated feet _______   Other ____

Atrophy: ____

Swelling: ____

Special Tests: ____

____

Mapping Palpation on Body Chart

X = trigger points   0 = tender points   B = taut bands

Grading Tender Points

1 = tenderness to 4 kg pressure (blanches therapist's fingernail bed)
2 = tenderness and wincing or moving away from 4 kg pressure
3 = jump sign or sharp withdrawal from 4 kg pressure
4 = client cannot allow therapist to touch

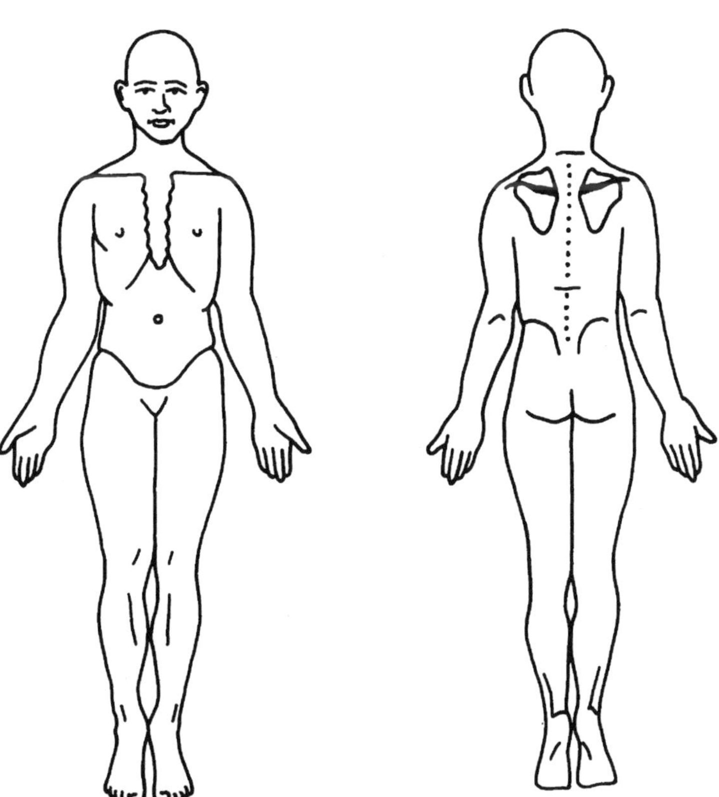

Education

Be positive when working with clients with FS and offer them hope. Many people with FS present to the physical therapist initially with a pessimistic outlook on treatment. Some of this attitude has to do with the years of trying to find a diagnosis and treatment. Many clients have come to view medical professionals negatively because they have spent so much energy and money and have received so little help. When they have finally found a diagnosis, they are told that there is no cure. They are thirsty for facts about FS. You must be straightforward with your clients and tell them that the body of knowledge about FS is incomplete at this time. As a result, there are no final answers to many of the questions they may have although there is a lot of hope to be found in current research. Be prepared to give them as much information as possible because education and understanding are always critical in clients' rehabilitation and self-care. Assure the client that you will utilize the available information to the best of your ability and if the client will do the same, there will be improvement in the level of pain and function.

There are several paradoxes in FS that may often confuse the client. For instance, we tell the client that one of the most helpful tools we have in dealing with FS is exercise. Most clients find this difficult to accept because they have tried exercise and it made them feel worse. For these clients you will need to explain that they probably were doing too much too soon. They need to start out more gradually. Other clients are perplexed that we are suggesting that they need to exercise when they have been very physically active for years. These are the people who either have the wrong diagnosis or who have overused their bodies to such an extent that the stresses and strains became unbalanced with the needed healing and repair. In other words, they were doing too much for too long. They have probably experienced excessive microtrauma and excessive fatigue. If the person also has a genetic predisposition to FS, the combination of these factors may be enough to set the syndrome in motion. We know that about 80% of FS patients are aerobically unfit. The other 20% are seeming paradoxes, including the types of people who have exercised vigorously for a long time.

Individuals with FS often complain that they feel like guinea pigs because the physician has tried medication after medication with them. In order to reassure clients, you need to understand that trial and error with medication, within a certain range, is the only method available to physicians at this point. Physicians are usually doing the best they can and are not indiscriminately trying one thing and then another. It is important to acquaint yourself with the medications that are currently used to treat FS so that you can help the patient become knowledgeable about treatment methods.

Another fear that clients express quite often is that the physician thinks their symptoms are "all in their heads" because they have been asked to take an antidepressant. Being aware that amitriptyline (elavil) is an antidepressant only when taken in higher dosages than the 10 to 75 milligrams per night that people with FS take will help you to reassure your clients that the symptoms are not imagined. The physician uses the antidepressant drug in a manner that has been shown through valid research to be effective for improved sleep and decreased pain in a majority of people who suffer from FS. Your explanation of the purpose of these medications will help to set the client's mind at ease.

Discussing clients' fear that their symptoms are imagined might be a good opportunity for you to bring up the possibility of the client finding a professional counselor who is well versed in FS. Professional counseling is another tool to help people cope with the chronic nature of the syndrome. It becomes difficult, if not impossible, to maintain relationships and perform daily activities while dealing with chronic pain as well as a fear of the unknown. Assisting your client to learn coping tools as well as physical tools provided by physical therapy can usually help the client achieve greater improvement.

A psychologist can offer a host of coping tools, including biofeedback, guided imagery, and stress management techniques. There is no denying that a strong interaction exists between the mind and body. Encourage your clients to look at the positive aspect of that interaction and utilize it to their benefit. In other words, reap the benefits of relaxation techniques, visualization, and positive thinking. We know that a physical body that is ill can facilitate a mental illness (usually reactive depression). By the same token, a strong, healthy mental attitude can help in restoring physical health.

To strengthen the idea that finding a counselor is helpful for the client, point out that programs in which several facets of the syndrome are addressed concurrently have been very successful (Bennett et al. 1991). Very few people are fortunate enough to have access to such multi-dimensional FS treatment programs, so we must simulate the concept as best we can.

Many times clients begin to doubt themselves and wonder if other people are correct when they say that the symptoms are "all in their heads." A support group is one of the best remedies for that self-doubt. Urge your client to attend such a group. If you do not know of such a group, call the local Arthritis Foundation to find out whether they are offering one. Another great source of information on support groups around the country is the *Fibromyalgia Network* newsletter. If there is a self-help directory published in your area, you might find an FS organization listed there. If no such group is available in your area, consider starting one yourself. You will learn a lot from the participants and you will be warmly rewarded by helping to fill this great need (see pages 101 to 102 for information on starting a support group).

Have some printed information available to send home with the client after the first visit with you. It is important for individuals with FS to have the opportunity to read and learn more about the syndrome and they will be reassured to know that research is ongoing. By reviewing the materials, the client's family will also have the opportunity to learn more about FS, which will help to validate the problems to the client's family, as well as to the client. Also, knowledge about the syndrome gives the individual an increased sense of control and mastery over life with FS.

There is so much literature available that it may be difficult to decide what to include in this initial information packet. Some suggestions of items to include are:

- articles describing the syndrome
- summaries of recent research findings
- a list of helpful hints on coping and pain management
- a chart to guide a person in determining the proper level of aerobic exercise
- information about psychological help
- information about local support groups and organizations
- a reading list of materials about FS

As a therapist, here are a few other suggestions for information that might be helpful to have in your files:

1. You can find many research articles by reading bibliographies of works written about FS. Usually, you can order copies of the articles from the medical library of a nearby hospital or directly from the author. If your clients are interested in reading these, you might lend your articles to them or suggest they order their own copies.

2. *The Journal of Musculoskeletal Pain* published by Haworth Press is an excellent new resource comprised of articles written primarily by FS researchers. (See page 103 for the address.)

3. *Fibromyalgia Network,* published by Health Information Network, Inc., Tucson, Arizona, is a user-friendly newsletter that reports on recent findings from research and on seminars that focus on FS and CFS. This company also provides information about active support groups around the country and publishes brochures about FS that you may find helpful. (See page 103 for the address.)

4. *When Muscle Pain Won't Go Away* is a paperback book published by Taylor Publishing Company. The book detailing FS was written by a patient, Gayle Backstrom, in association with her rheumatologist, Dr. Bernard R. Rubin. It is a useful resource to recommend to clients because it is well written and includes thorough listings of related resources and helpful organizations. It is available in most bookstores.

5. *Caring for Your Wife in Sickness and in Health* by Richard H. Dominguez, M.D., is published by Discovery House Publishers, P.O. Box 3566, Grand Rapids, MI 49501-3566, Phone: 1-800-653-8333. This book contains practical, workable, and honest suggestions for coping with a chronic illness. It is a particularly helpful resource for spouses.

In addition, the information on pages 70, 71, 90, and 92 is helpful to provide for clients.

Clinical Treatment

It is necessary to begin this section with a caveat: Not all of the following ideas for treatment have been proven by research. They have been developed through my own clinical experiences in conjunction with information gleaned from researchers and other therapists and from physical therapy training. It is not intended that this collection of ideas be viewed as final or complete. There is still a lot to learn.

A few general comments are in order before considering the suggested protocol.

1. As far as we know at this time, FS is a condition that will stay with the individual for a lifetime. This means that the person with FS will not be back to normal after a specified number of physical therapy treatments. If the physician or insurance company has specified the number of treatments the individual may receive, it is up to you to use those treatments to your client's best benefit. Usually, the best way to maximize the benefits from therapy is to spread out the appointments. This allows your client adequate time to incorporate the exercises and other tools that you teach at each session in order to better utilize those that you will teach at the next session. FS is a chronic condition and will usually require months of working with the tools you teach in order to realize change. A lot of this work will probably be done by your client outside the clinic.

2. It is the nature of people with FS to adapt to exercise slowly. One of the most common mistakes in starting clients with FS on an exercise program seems to be too much, too soon, which often causes a worsening of their symptoms. When this happens, it becomes much more difficult to convince the person that exercise is beneficial. Begin at a low level in terms of repetitions and resistance. For example, many people with FS need to begin with three repetitions of an exercise using no resistance.

3. Modalities have a definite place in the treatment of people with FS in helping to calm down the pain during a severe flaring of symptoms. In this protocol, modalities are used but the role of modalities, other than moist heat, is downplayed because clients need to learn tools they can use at home in order to manage the FS on their own as much as possible. They probably will not have access to clinical modalities, such as ultrasound, on an ongoing basis so it would not be helpful to allow clients to rely on them.

4. Isometric exercise is not used in this protocol because isometric contractions cause a decrease in blood flow of up to 40% and people with FS seem to have some microcirculation disturbance already. This approach is supported by Klug, McAuley, and Clark (1989), who state that "If oxygenation is indeed a problem in the muscle tissue of patients with fibrositis, use of this type of exercise (isometric) may only aggravate this difficulty. Moreover, if the cardiovascular or skeletal muscle adaptations that occur as a result of aerobic training prove to be beneficial in fibrositis, isometric exercise would be of

little benefit as none of the changes result from this type of training." Avoidance of isometrics seems to be indicated in those patients who also have mitral valve prolapse (MVP) because "recent studies have shown that sudden blood pressure changes are associated with this type of activity, so isometric exercises may be an unwise choice for the MVP patient, who may already have problems with unstable blood pressure" (Frederickson 1988).

Similarly, eccentric exercises are largely avoided because they are implicated in delayed onset of muscle soreness and clients with FS do not appreciate more muscle pain than they already have. Klug, McAuley, and Clark (1989) suggest that "swimming and cycling at a low work load might be modes of choice over jogging because of the difference in the percentage of total contractions that are eccentric." If your client's job (recreation) necessitates a lot of eccentric contraction, discuss the importance of relaxing those muscle groups frequently.

5. *Subtle* is a key word for describing the approach to treating people with FS, whether you are designing the exercise program, applying soft tissue massage, or choosing which modality to use. A key phrase is "lots of little bits" in regard to the frequency of soft tissue work and of strengthening exercises.

6. Always treat bilaterally. You will almost always find that tender/trigger points occur symmetrically on both sides of the body, despite the fact that only one side might be symptomatic at the time of evaluation.

7. Remind the client that the main goal of treatment is to increase function. The increase in function is the yardstick by which to measure improvement because sometimes a client's pain level seems to be unchanged, yet the client is able to function better. The secondary goal is to decrease pain. Decreasing pain is definitely important, but increasing function remains the primary goal.

8. The second main goal of treatment relates to increasing function and involves teaching the client to become the manager of the syndrome. We can help clients accomplish this goal through the education we impart and the tools (techniques) for home use that we share. Many clients learn to use tools that help them when the muscle pain begins and to prevent it from worsening.

9. Keep listening. By taking the time to listen, you will continue to learn about the specific precipitating factors, the pain pattern, and even past history. This knowledge will doubtless assist you in guiding your client to manage the symptoms. Each client with fibromyalgia exhibits a specific pattern of the syndrome that is not exactly like that of any other client. Also, by continuing to listen, you reassure your client, which is critical for developing a healing relationship. Finally, listening to all of your clients with FS will help educate you about this still mysterious and fascinating medical condition.

Protocol

The following protocol is a guideline only, as is any good protocol. Your initial evaluation of the client will determine where in the protocol you will begin. Progression is dictated by the client's tolerance and your therapeutic discretion.

STAGE 1

Scope

Stage 1 will probably encompass one to four sessions. The exact number of sessions will depend on the length of each session, the client's knowledge of FS, and the client's level of pain. The interval between sessions will be determined by the acuteness of the client's pain and the amount of information covered at each session. For instance, if the client has acute pain and needs more help initially from modalities, then the first few sessions will probably be closer together than the last few sessions. If the client has already found helpful resources and has networked with others who have FS, then the time you spend on education will be reduced compared to the time you would spend with someone who has recently been diagnosed and is completely puzzled or even hostile.

The tools presented in Stage 1 do not need to be used or taught within a certain time frame or performed in any particular order. You and your client will quickly recognize which ones are the most effective. The goal of Stage 1 is to prepare the client and the client's muscles for exercising.

Try to limit actual treatment on the first day to only a few of these Stage 1 tools because the client will have already undergone an evaluation during this visit and received a lot of new information to absorb. Warn the client that some increased soreness may result from the evaluation. Hopefully, you have been careful enough to keep this discomfort to a minimum. Plan to see the client again in two or three days.

Stretching (Muscle Lengthening)

There are three reasons for stretching exercises for clients with FS:

1. to help correct postural imbalances

2. to relieve pain from trigger/tender points

3. to help deactivate the tender/trigger points

Teach slow, sustained, gentle stretches for the appropriate muscles according to your initial evaluation of flexibility and trigger point location. Remind the client that only discomfort, not pain, should be felt while stretching. If the client tries to stretch more forcefully, which may result in pain, the muscles will try to guard and cause increased tension rather than allow the desired lengthening. The following are some of the most common stretches that you are likely to teach. Remember to present only a few at each session.

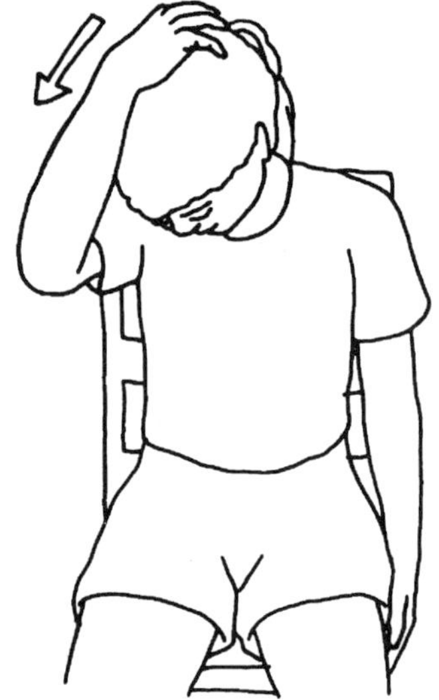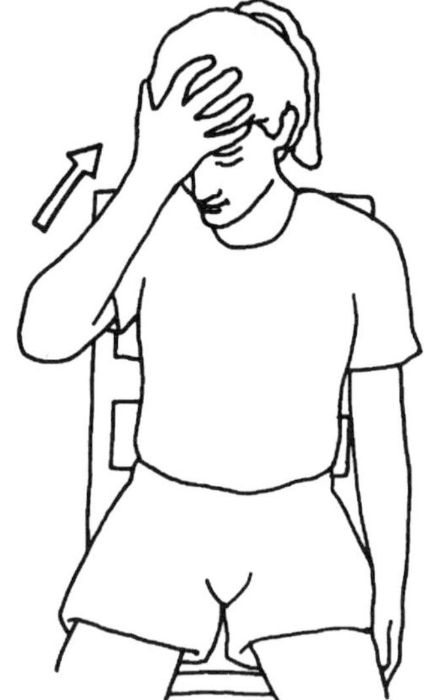

Figure 3. **Levator Scapula Stretch: Position 1**

Figure 4. **Levator Scapula Stretch Release: Position 2**

Stretching the levator scapulae is often needed. Ask the client to look toward one knee and use the ipsilateral hand to apply overpressure. Remind the client to hold the stretch for a sustained time (about 30 seconds if tolerated). Ask the client to rotate the head during this stretch to find the angle that is the tightest. Then use that angle for the next stretch. Figure 4 demonstrates using the arm and hand to return the head to neutral following the stretch, which allows the levator scapula muscle fibers to remain relatively lengthened by not calling on them to contract to help return the head to neutral.

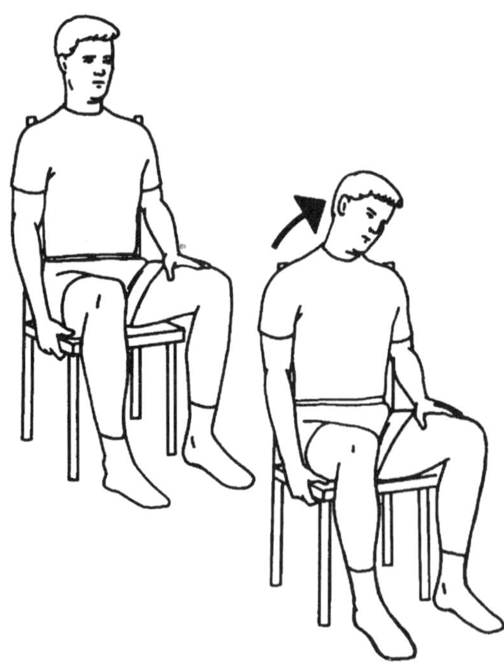

Figure 5. **Upper Trapezius Stretch**

Have the client anchor one hand by holding on to the chair seat. The client then leans to the opposite side letting the neck sidebend in that direction. As in the last stretch, you may have the client help the head return to neutral by using the hand to push it rather than contracting the upper trapezius.

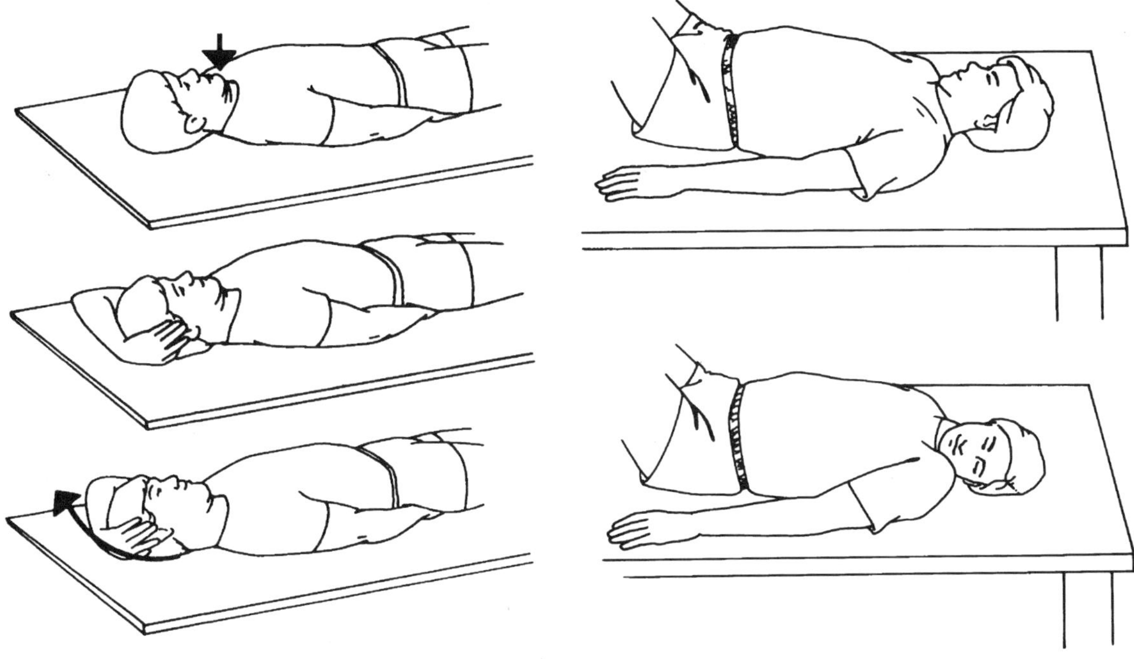

Figure 6. Neck Lateral Flexor Stretch

Figure 7. Neck Rotation

These two stretches are often most effective when done in the supine position as shown. Overpressure given by the client can be used with neck rotation as well as neck lateral flexion.

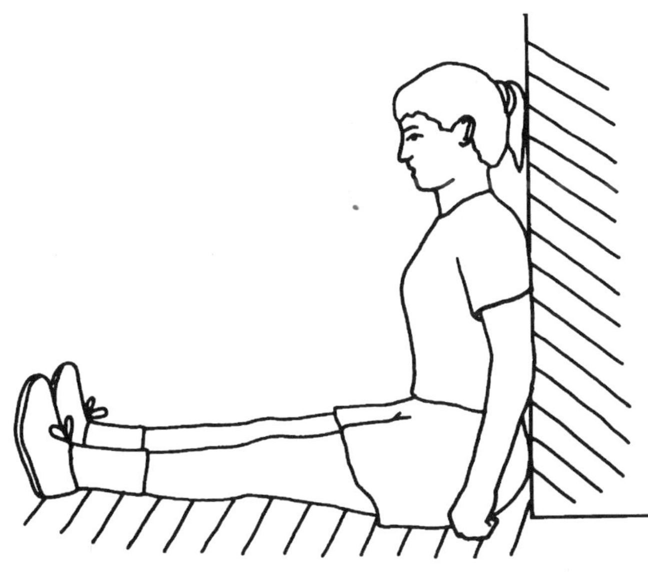

Figure 8. Hamstring Stretch

This is a safe, easy, and adequate way to stretch the hamstring muscles. Have the client sit so that the entire back is touching the wall. Then have the client straighten the legs while keeping the knees pointed upward.

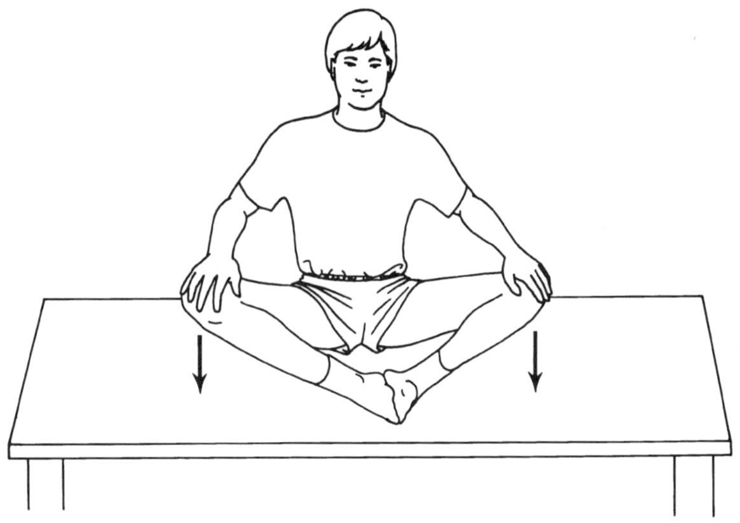

***Figure 9.* Adductor Stretch**

Have the client sit against a wall or firm piece of furniture and bring the soles of the feet together. Gently apply downward pressure on the knees. Hold for 15-30 seconds.

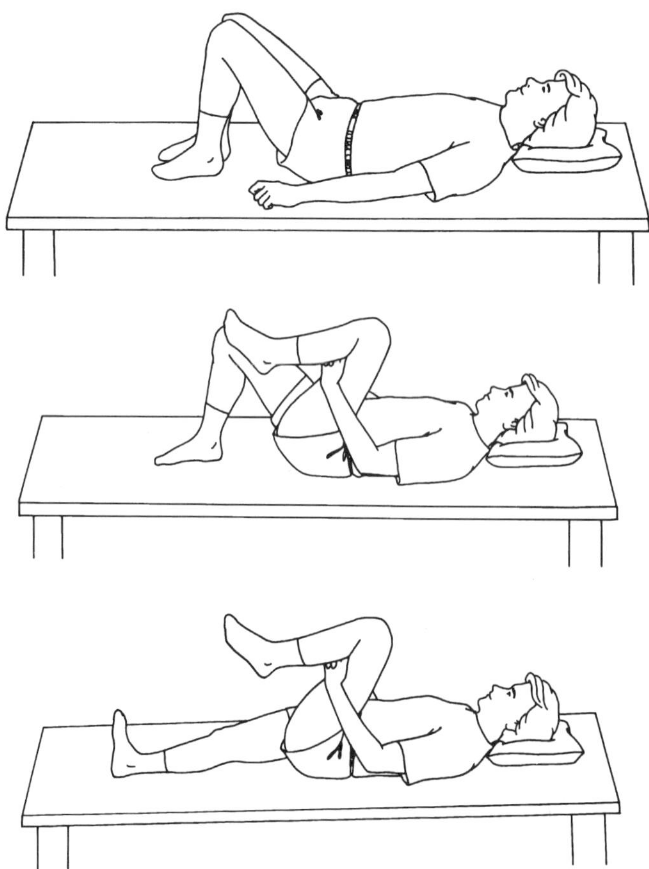

***Figure 10.* Single Knee to Chest Stretch for the Low Back and Hip Area**

While lying on the back, the client pulls one knee toward the chest until stretching is felt and holds to tolerance. Repeat with the other leg.

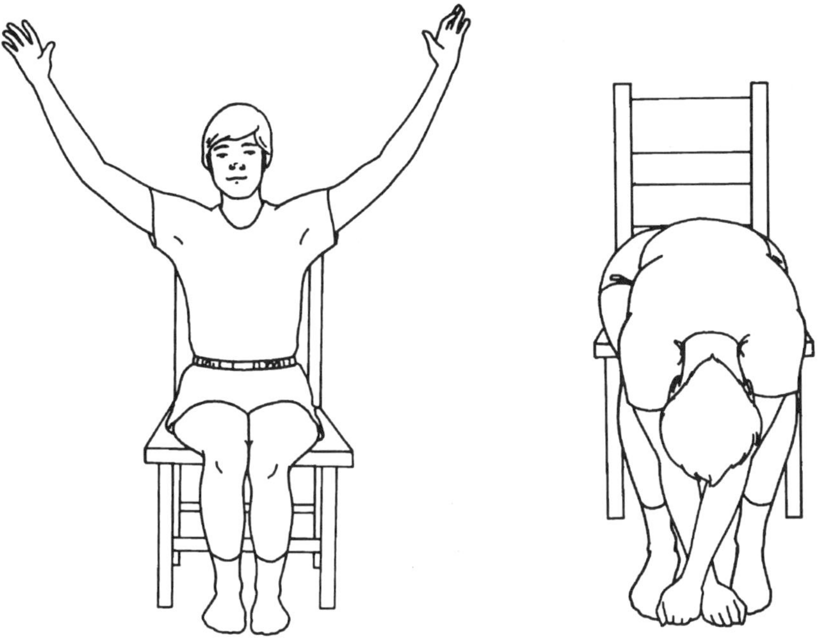

Figure 11. **Low Back Stretch**

While the client is seated, have the client breathe in through the nose while raising the arms over head then breathe out while bending forward. The feet can be placed farther from the body and the same process repeated. This allows stretching lower in the back.

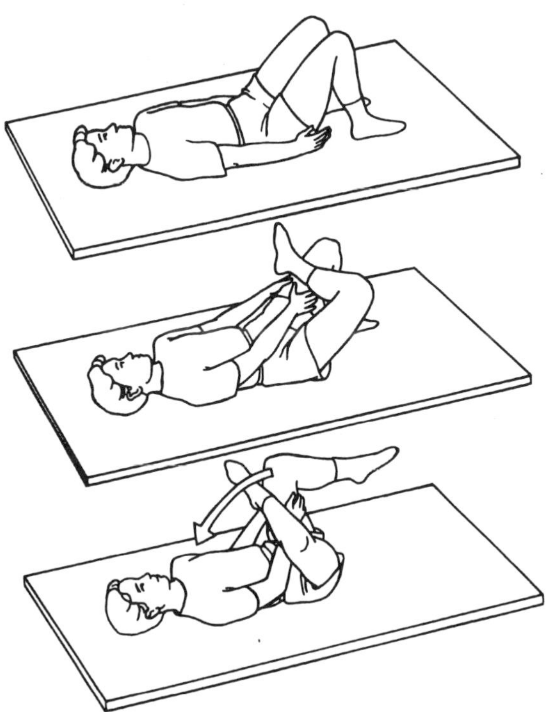

Figure 12. **Hip Internal (Medial) Rotator and Extensor Stretch**

Ask the client to lie on the back with knees bent and bring the right ankle to the left thigh. Prompt the client to put both hands around the left thigh and pull it toward the body. The stretch will be felt in the right hip. Then have the client switch legs and stretch the left hip.

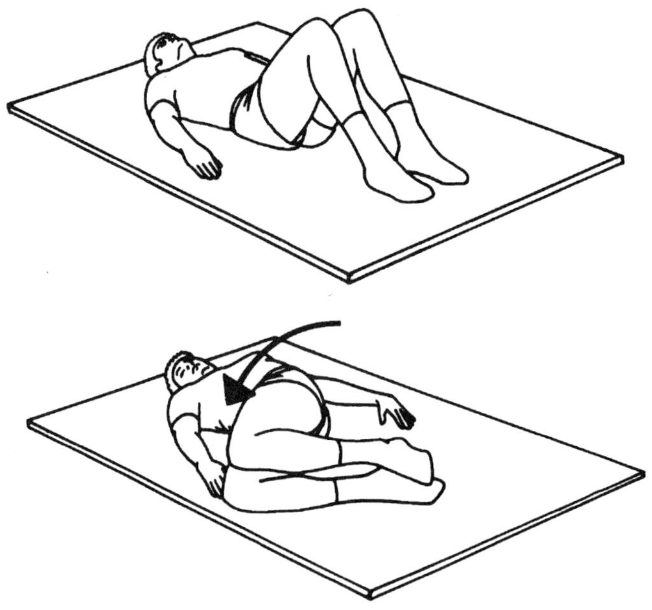

Figure 13. **Trunk Stretch**

Have the client lie on the back and bend the knees. The client will move the knees to one side and keep the shoulders down on the surface. After holding for 15 to 20 seconds, the client slowly brings the knees back up, moves them to the other side, and stretches again. The feet can be placed farther away from the body and the same process repeated. This allows for stretching lower in the back.

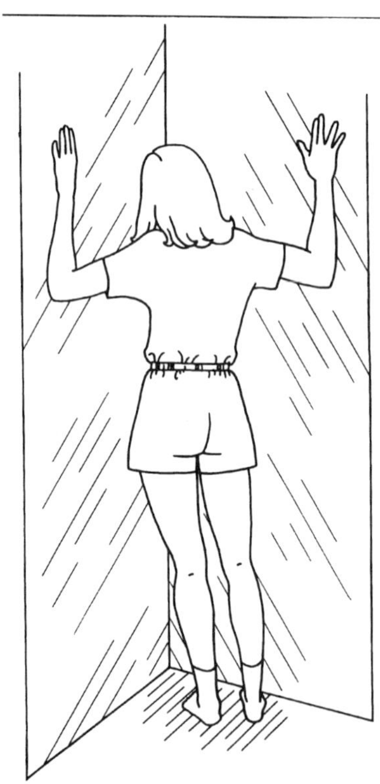

Figure 14. **Pectoralis Stretch (Corner Stretch)**

The client stands in a corner with the forearms on the wall. Ask the client to lean the chest toward the corner and hold the stretch for 15 to 20 seconds. Suggest that the client try the stretch with the hands at various heights.

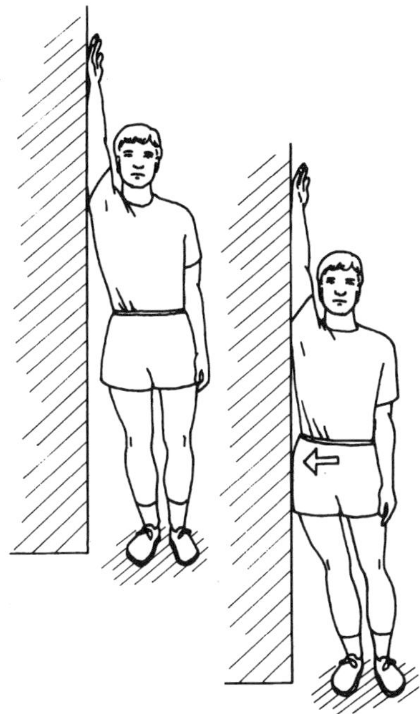

Have the client stand with the right side of the body 12″ from the wall. Prompt the client to tighten the abdominals then place the right arm against the wall and lean the right hip toward the wall. The stretch should be held for 15 to 20 seconds and repeated several times. Have the client turn around and stretch the left side.

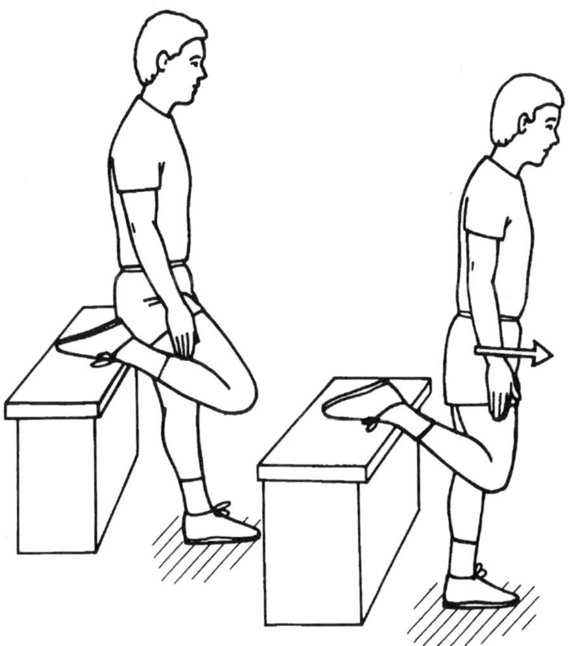

Position the client in front of a table or bench. Ask the client to place the right foot on the table while keeping the back straight and the abdominals tightened. The client should lean the trunk forward to feel the stretch on the front of the right thigh. Repeat with the left leg.

HOT TIPS
for People with Fibromyalgia

✔ Stay warm and avoid drafts. Long underwear made of silk is great—warm, yet very lightweight. Avoid sitting near a cold air return.

✔ Use your headrest while in the car.

✔ Try a heat massager to relieve pain.

✔ Remember to **HALT:** don't let yourself get too **H**ungry, **A**ngry, **L**onely, or **T**ired.

✔ Decrease stress in your life.

✔ Try to **PACE** yourself. **P**repare ahead. **A**llow time for relaxation. **C**hange work position often. **E**verybody pitch in.

✔ Don't hold the phone receiver between your head and shoulder.

✔ Avoid carrying a shoulder bag.

✔ Avoid working overhead; for instance, when painting your house or trimming tall bushes.

✔ Use a tennis ball against the wall or floor to massage your own back, or try leaning into a doorjamb to apply compression to your trigger points.

✔ Avoid caffeine and tobacco.

✔ Use an external support (brace or towel roll) when you are tired but **must** keep going.

✔ Fidget!

✔ Drink lots of water.

✔ Sleep with a towel roll around your neck and/or waist.

✔ Avoid tasks that require more strength than you currently possess, such as lifting heavy groceries or walking a large dog.

✔ Do some gentle arm and neck range of motion movements before you get out of bed.

✔ Use moist heat, such as a shower or jacuzzi, or a moist heating pad.

✔ When an irritating situation arises, slow down your breathing to help you remain calm.

✔ Learn a relaxation technique.

✔ Remember that the key word is "subtle" for your stretching and exercise routines.

✔ Be careful when lifting small children.

Adapted with permission from: SportsMed Orthopaedics and Rehabilitation (Wheaton Orthopaedics, Ltd.) Carol Stream, IL.

AEROBIC WORKOUTS
for People with Fibromyalgia

For an effective aerobic workout, you are typically instructed to find your target heart rate (THR) in beats per minute by using the following formula:

220 minus your age

For example, for a 48-year-old person: 220 - 48 = 172

Then find 70% to 80% of that number—70% for an intermediate level of aerobic fitness and up to 85% for an advanced level.

Continuing the example above: 70% x 172 = 120.4

so, the THR is 120 beats per minute

The following chart shows the target rates at the intermediate and advanced levels.

Target Heart Rates

Age (years)	70% (intermediate level)	85% (advanced level)	Maximum Attainable Heart Rate
25	140	170	200
30	136	169	194
35	132	160	186
40	128	155	182
45	124	150	176
50	119	145	171
55	115	140	165
60	111	135	159
65	107	130	153

But what should you do if you are a beginner? It is particularly important for people with fibromyalgia to ask that question. About 80% of people with FS are deconditioned and aerobically unfit. In such a situation, the intensity level should be decreased to approximately 50% or 60% of your maximum heart rate. For the previous example involving a 48-year-old person, the THR would be reduced from 172 at 70% to 86 or 103 beats per minute at 50% or 60%, respectively.

People with FS often find they do not tolerate aerobic exercise and report increased pain for days afterward. Therefore, people with FS are understandably hesitant to pursue aerobic exercise. This situation can be remedied by altering other factors, such as the frequency and duration of the aerobic exercise. Below is a formula for finding the appropriate training intensity for each week. Ideally, training intensity for one week should equal 42 in order to attain aerobic fitness.

training intensity = intensity (percent) X frequency (sessions per week) X duration (minutes per session)

For example, each of the following weekly schedules yields a training intensity of 42:

50% X 3 sessions/week X 28 minutes/session = 42

50% X 4 sessions/week X 21 minutes/session = 42

60% X 4 sessions/week X 17.5 minutes/session = 42

60% X 5 sessions/week X 14 minutes/session = 42

Prior to beginning an aerobic exercise program, you should first calculate your target heart rate using the formula at the top of the page and the percentage of intensity that is right for you. Then calculate your training intensity program using the formula above. If you find that you tolerate exercise better in smaller amounts of time and need to keep the percentage of intensity fairly low, you might choose a program like the fourth example given above. Following this schedule, you will get your heart rate up to your THR and maintain it for 14 minutes. You will need to exercise at this intensity 5 times each week.

Adapted with permission from: SportsMed Orthopaedics and Rehabilitation (Wheaton Orthopaedics, Ltd.) Carol Stream, IL.

Modalities

Moist heat. Moist heat almost universally provides some measure of relief for people with FS. There are many options available commercially so clients have no trouble following through with this tool. It can be used simply to relieve pain or to facilitate stretching. Some stretches can safely be performed by the client in the moist heat of a shower. Research by Hong and colleagues (1993) has shown that hydrocollator packs cause a significant elevation in pain threshold thereby decreasing clients' pain. Pain was measured with an algometer in this study.

Ultrasound. This modality is a good option for clients with deep-seated or long-standing soft tissue changes. A study by Hong and colleagues (1993) has proven that its use affected a significant elevation in the patients' pain threshold. Hong and his colleagues used 1.2-1.5 watts/cm^2 for 5 minutes with slow, circular movement of the sound head. Travell and Simons (1983) indicate that low-intensity ultrasound deactivates trigger points. In their manual, they also offer two suggestions for ultrasound use. First, the intensity should be at 0.5 watts/cm^2 moving the sound head in a slow, circular motion over the trigger point. In the second technique, the intensity is increased to 1.5 watts/cm^2, unless the pain level requires stopping at a lower intensity. If there is pain, then the power is reduced to half of the maximum intensity that was reached. In a few minutes, the therapist gradually increases the intensity until the maximum (up to 1.5 watts/cm^2) has been reached comfortably. The authors do not suggest any specific duration of treatment. Another author (Starlanyl 1994) found that using sine-wave ultrasound with electrostimulation was effective therapeutically as well as diagnostically in dealing with tender points.

Stretch and spray. The combination of stretching the affected muscle and applying Fluori-Methane spray (Gebauer Chemical Company, Cleveland, Ohio, 44104) in a sweeping fashion in line with the fibers of the affected muscle has been shown by Hong and colleagues (1993) to be more effective than thermotherapy. Travell and Simons (1983) have promoted this technique and emphasized the "stretch" aspect. They teach the therapist to direct the spray in the direction of referred pain first and then to spray throughout the referred pain pattern for that particular trigger point. Charts in their books illustrate these patterns. The can should be held at a 30-degree angle to the skin and about 18 inches away from the client. Make two or three slow sweeps with the spray, gently stretching the involved muscle. Repeat the cycle several times. The rapid evaporation of the spray causes cooling of the stream so that it cools superficial tissues and facilitates stretching of the muscle, presumably by affecting skin afferent nerves (Travell and Simons 1983). It is recommended that the skin be warmed between stretches and at the end of the treatment. This routine can become part of a client's home program if there is someone at home who is willing to help.

Recently, information about the ill effects of fluorocarbons on the atmosphere have led to a search for a new vapocoolant spray. In the meantime, Travell and Simons (1992) have suggested an alternative technique called *intermittent cold with stretch.* Stroking with ice is an effective substitute for the spray, but you must keep drying the skin because "dampness reduces the rate of the change in skin

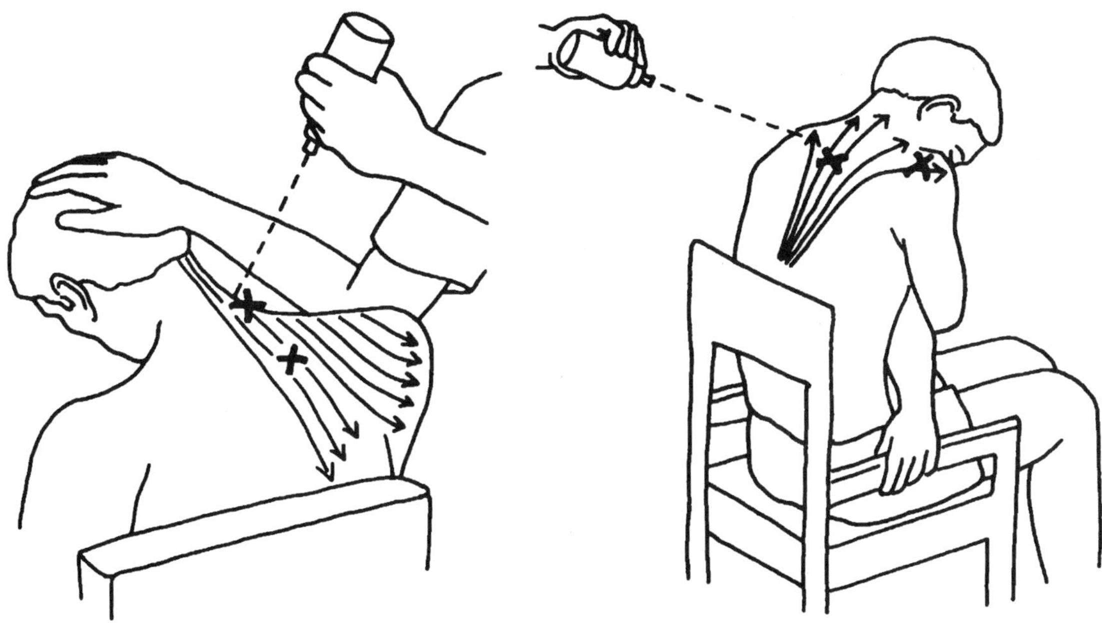

Figure 17. Stretch and Spray Technique   **Figure 18.** Stretch and Spray Technique

The X's in these illustrations indicate the location of trigger points in these muscles.

temperature produced by the ice-stroking. Wetness also prolongs and diffuses the cooling effect, which delays rewarming of the skin." The authors warned against cooling the underlying musculature. Only the skin should be cooled in this technique.

Microcurrent. Some patients have reported good relief with the clinical use of microcurrent. It is not clear whether the effectiveness of the treatment is related to electrode placement or simply the differences among people with fibromyalgia. The manufacturer's information claims that microcurrent boosts ATP. If this actually happens, then it would explain microcurrent's efficacy in some clients.

Biofeedback. Biofeedback can be used very effectively to help clients realize that their muscles are not relaxed when they believe that they are relaxed. It can also be used to help them learn how to maintain relaxation in the positions they must assume for performing their work or during recreation. The biofeedback modality can also be used to re-educate a muscle that has stopped performing its normal function. A study in which EMG biofeedback was used with people with FS found that after 15 sessions they experienced fewer tender points, decreased pain, and decreased morning stiffness (Ferraccioli et al. 1987). They also found that there was no placebo effect. The only people who experienced benefits were those in the true biofeedback situation.

Transcutaneous electrical nerve stimulation (TENS), acupuncture, application of blistering agent (or capsaicin), dry needling. Some clients with FS have found varying degrees of relief with the use of these modalities. Melzack (1981) suggests that these are all methods of hyperstimulating an area in order to achieve analgesia.

A common term for this approach is *counterirritation.* In fact, Melzack (1981) claims responsibility for developing the approach of administering TENS at moderate to high intensity for brief periods of time (20 minutes). He conducted studies comparing this approach of using TENS with the use of acupuncture and found that the two approaches were basically equal in terms of effectiveness. Of course, the TENS modality outscored acupuncture for practicality and noninvasiveness. Melzack believes that the gate control theory explains the efficacy of hyperstimulation analgesia. When the hyperstimulating agent (TENS) acts on the small nerve fibers, it increases the input at the brainstem area, which has been dubbed the "central biasing mechanism." This barrage of input closes the gate so that other inputs from the body cannot get through the gate. This brief pain-free period allows the participant to move and work in normal physical patterns. Melzack suggests that these normal movements might help extend the pain-free window of time and prevent relapse into the abnormal neural activity.

Posture Awareness and Modifications

Your initial evaluation will have revealed any imbalances, poor habits, leg length discrepancy, or weaknesses that need to be altered. If there are several postural deviations to be corrected, begin with only one or two. This process will be no different than with any other client who needs postural correction. The goal is still neutral spine.

Some of the most frequently observed deviations are:

- forward head, usually accompanied by rounded shoulders
- asymmetry of scapulae, statically and dynamically

Suggestions for dealing with the forward head and rounded shoulders include the following.

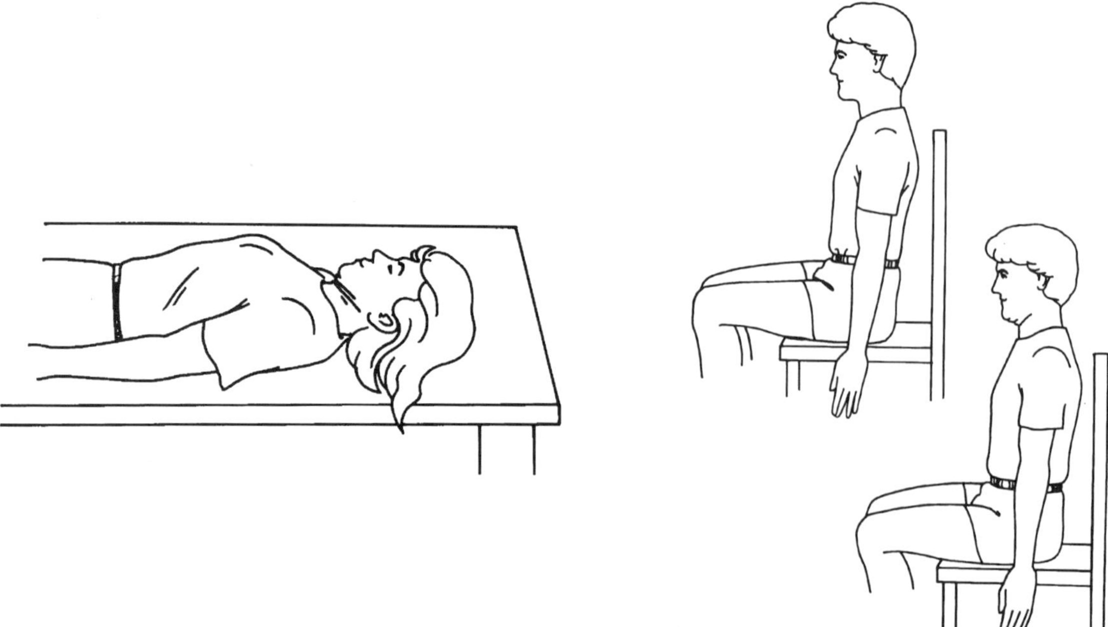

Figure 19. Neck Retraction, Supine

Figure 20. Neck Retraction, Straight

Remind the client to tuck the chin in and not tilt the head up or down. This is a horizontal motion.

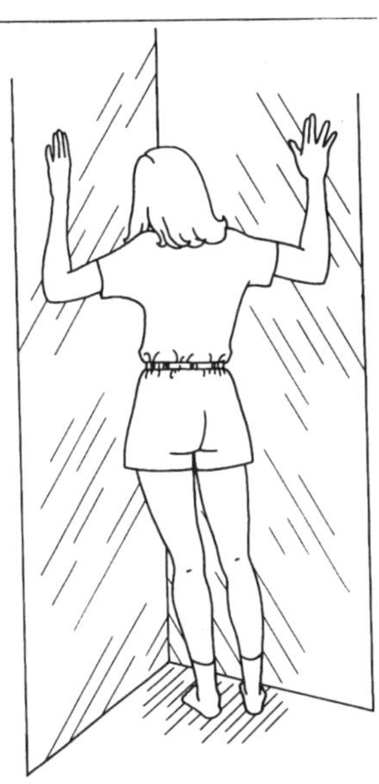

Figure 21. Pectoralis Stretches (Corner Stretch)

The client stands in a corner with the forearms on the wall. Ask the client to lean the chest toward the corner and hold the stretch for 15 to 20 seconds.

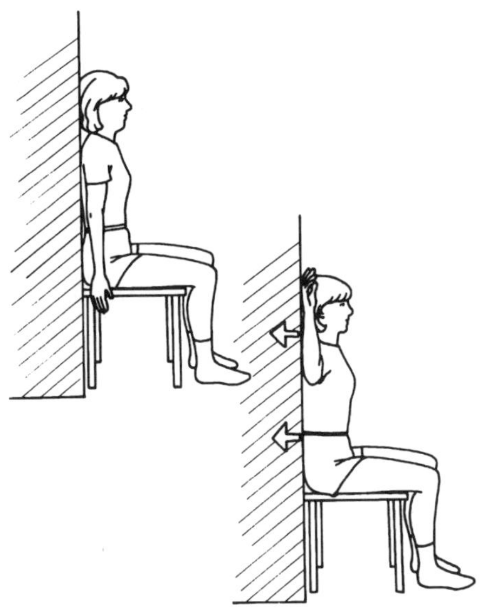

Figure 22. Scapula Retraction

Have the client sit with the back and head against a wall. The hands should be placed beside the head with the back of the arms touching the wall. Ask the client to press both the neck and back against the wall.

Suggestions for dealing with the poorly stabilized scapulae include strengthening the muscles that stabilize the scapulae (the middle and lower trapezius, serratus anterior, and rhomboids). Here are a few suggestions.

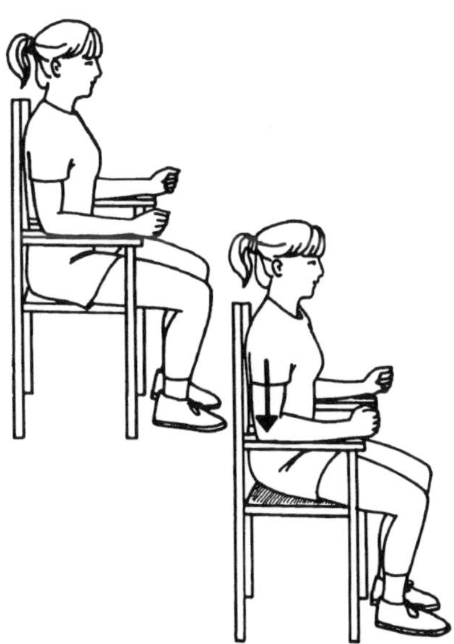

Figure 23. Scapula Retraction and Latissimus Strengthening

The client should be seated in a chair with the forearms on the arms of the chair. Have the client push the forearms down into the chair arms and squeeze the scapulae together.

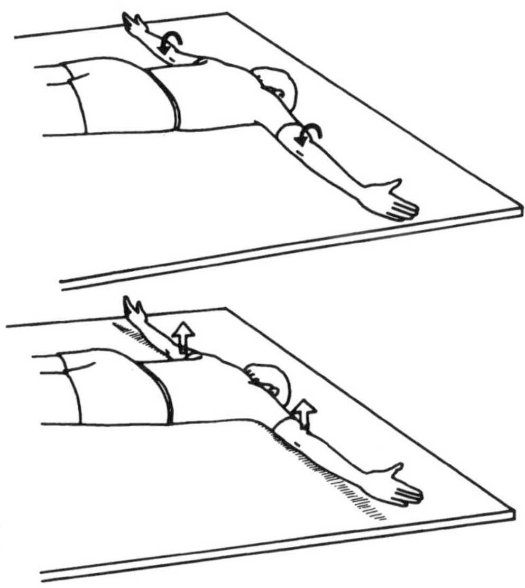

Figure 24. Further Strengthening of Scapular Muscles (Middle Trapezius)

Ask the client to lie on the stomach with arms out to the sides, parallel to the shoulders. The elbows should be straight and the thumbs up. Have the client pinch the shoulder blades together, raising the arms.

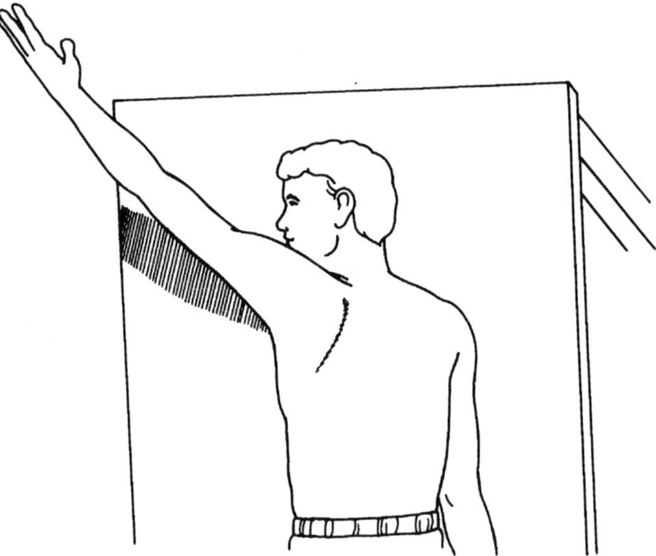

Figure 25. Further Strengthening of Scapular Muscles (Lower Trapezius)

Have the client lie on the stomach with the left arm overhead. Ask the client to move the left shoulder blade down and in toward the spine then raise the arm up, keeping elbow and hand level. Repeat with the other arm.

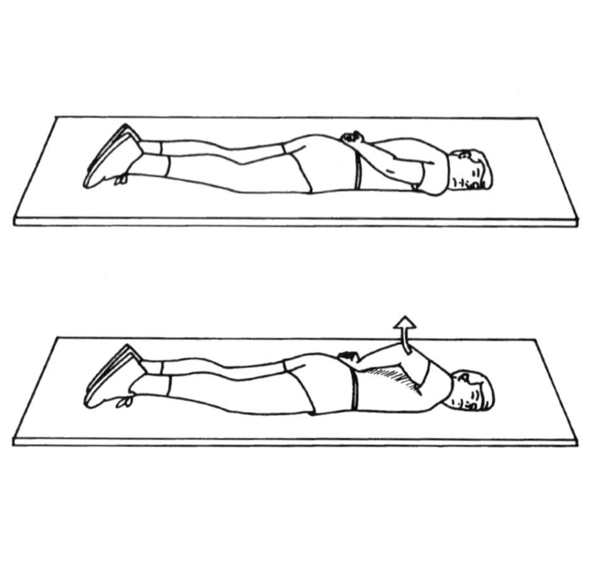

Figure 26. Scapula Retraction

Have the client lie on the stomach and place the right hand on the lower back. Ask the client to lift the elbow up and in while keeping the hand in place. Repeat with the other hand.

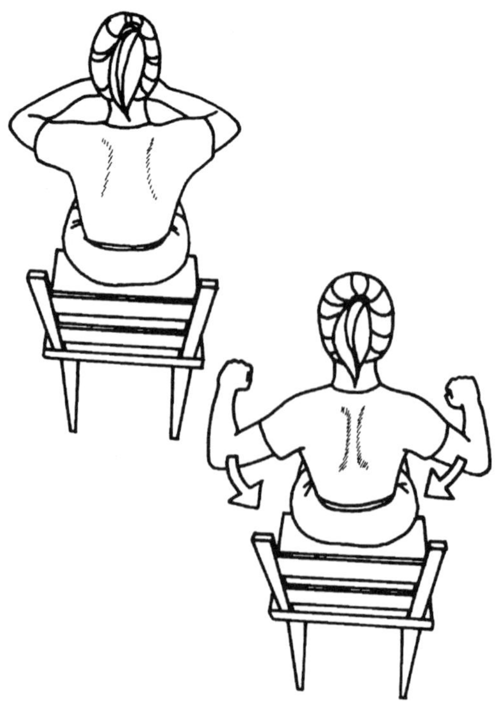

Figure 27. Seated Scapula Retraction

The client should be seated with arms at shoulder height and elbows bent. Prompt the client to pinch the shoulder blades together.

Many people are unable to actively recruit the lower trapezius at first so you will probably need to teach them how to do so in the sidelying position (see figure 28). Place the client's upper shoulder in external rotation and glide the scapula caudally and vertebrally. Teach the client to contract and hold in that position. You may need to add a little resistance at the acromion to help the client find the muscle.

When your client has grasped this lesson, work on it again in the upright position. Next teach your client to begin elevation of the shoulder, keeping the scapula motionless for the first 30 degrees.

This process is often expedited by the use of a biofeedback unit (see figure 29). Biofeedback can be used to re-educate the lower trapezius as well as to teach the upper trapezius to relax and stop overworking. Many times the upper trapezius is overworking and increasing its trigger point activity while the middle and lower trapezia are no longer doing their jobs. It is very important to correct this imbalance.

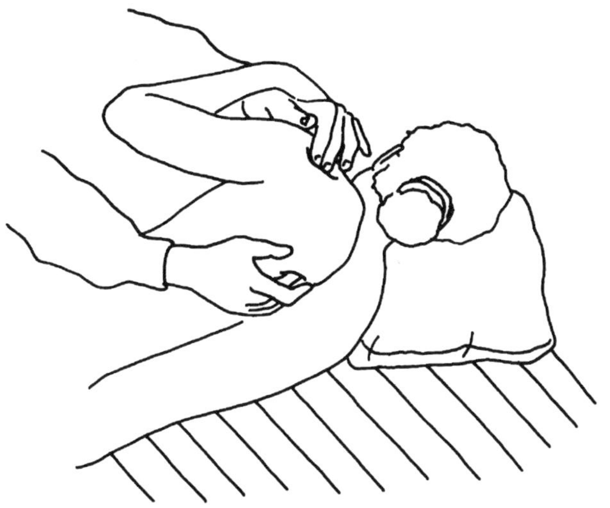

Figure 28. **Learning to Recruit the Lower Trapezius**

Note that the therapist's fingers are palpating the lower trapezius while the left hand is applying some resistance against the action of the lower trapezius. Also, the therapist's left forearm is supporting the client's arm in slight external rotation.

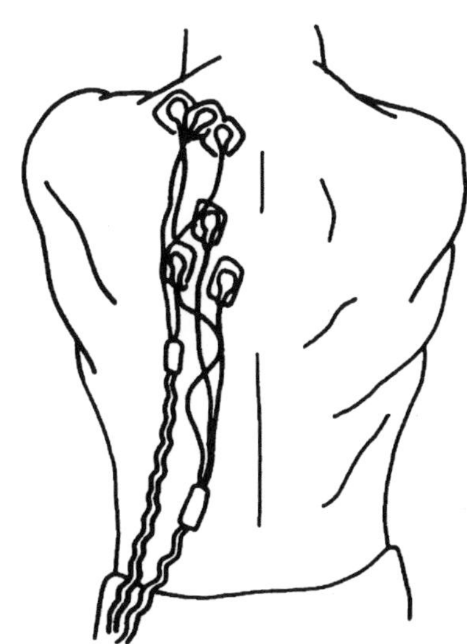

Figure 29. **Using Biofeedback for Reeducation**

This illustration shows the biofeedback setup with the electrodes on the lower trapezius giving feedback on the active recruitment of these fibers while the electrodes on the upper trapezius will report on the status of relaxation of these fibers. For this setup, you will need to use two separate biofeedback units or two separate channels on one unit.

Remember to correct sitting and sleeping postures at this time also. Many people spend most of their day sitting at their job and in front of the television. The most common sitting deviation is the forward flexed posture, or C-curve, which facilitates shoulder protraction. In an excellent article on sitting posture and its culpability in carpal tunnel syndrome, Zacharkow (1994) suggests that a lower thoracic support and a sacral support on the chair back be utilized. He states that this will affect elevation of the sternum, ribs, chest, and diaphragm, which will improve posture, relieve compression at the thoracic outlet, and facilitate the back extensors.

Occasionally, a few cues from you will be sufficient, but usually people need a more constant reminder such as the aforementioned supports. Sometimes you will need to help the client figure out how to alter the desk chair or the arrangement of objects on the desk.

If possible, find out the client's sleep position(s). Sometimes clients say they do not know how they sleep. Since sleeping position can make a difference in how people with FS feel when they awaken, teach them how to support their bodies well in the supine, sidelying, and prone positions, using extra pillows where necessary (see figures 31 and 32).

It is difficult to make the neck comfortable and relaxed in the prone position, so clients are probably better off if they avoid sleeping prone. If the client does not sleep prone, one of the most simple tools for providing support is a towel rolled lengthwise, wrapped around the neck, and tied in front with a string.

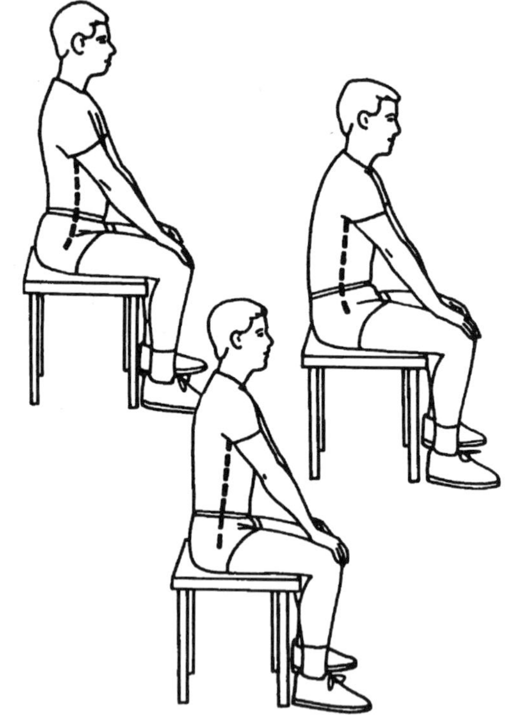

Figure 30. **Neutral Spine in Sitting**

Strive for neutral spine in sitting, which will require tightening of the abdominals.

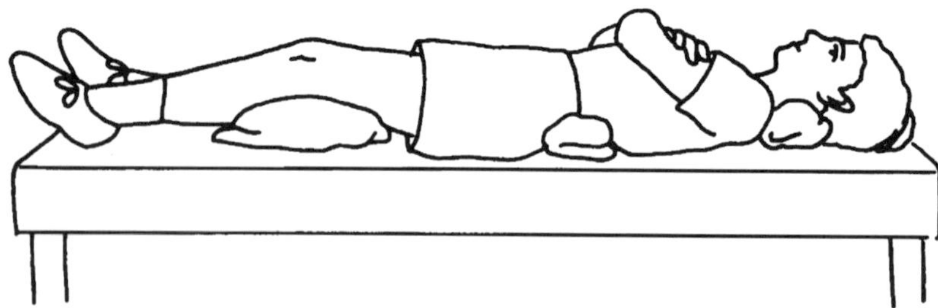

Figure 31. **Supported Sleep Position in Supine**

Note the positioning of pillows and towel rolls in this figure to support natural curves of the body.

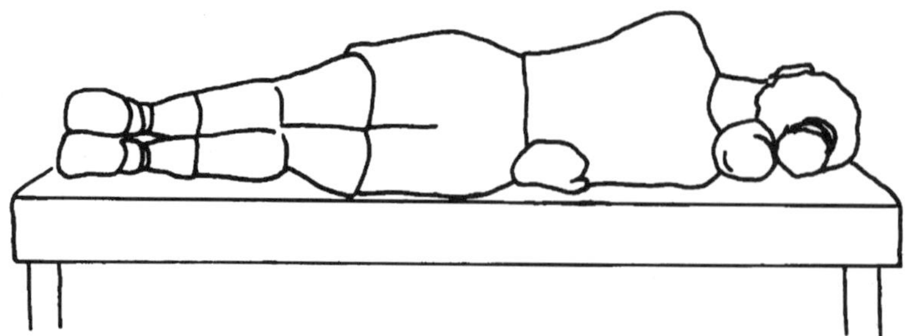

Figure 32. **Supported Sleep Position in Sidelying**

Note the use of rolls to support the spine. Many people find that adding a pillow between the knees is also necessary.

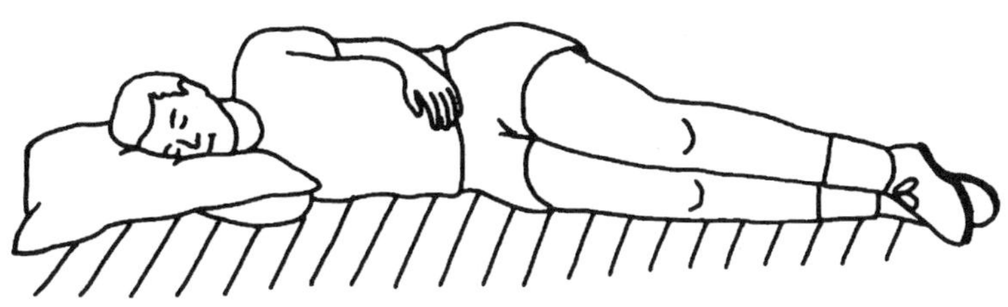

Figure 33. **Alternate Sleep Position in Sidelying**

This sidelying sleep position is also helpful because it allows the scapulae to rest in anatomical position and allows the posterior muscles to rest in a neutral position. Notice the top arm is in slight shoulder extension.

You will need to try a few different towels in order to find the best diameter so that the towel roll helps to support the neck and provides the most comfort. Many clients have reported improvement in morning stiffness when they use this inexpensive, custom-made tool.

Soft Tissue Mobilization

A variety of massage techniques can be used to effect temporary pain relief in the muscles of your clients with FS. Several therapeutic benefits can be derived from massage, such as increasing the blood flow and warming, so massage in general can be helpful.

In order to effect a longer-lasting benefit for people with FS, a technique called *ischemic compression* described by Travell and Simons (1983) may be used. This technique requires sustained (20 seconds to 1 minute) and gradually increasing pressure directly on a trigger point in an attempt to deactivate the trigger point (see figure 34, page 80).

Prior to applying pressure, the involved muscle should be placed on a stretch. The process is uncomfortable (often described by patients as "It's a good hurt") but should not be so uncomfortable that muscle guarding occurs. In that case, your treatment will be ineffective. Your treatment will also be worthless if you are not accurate about pinpointing the trigger point. Let the patient guide you verbally.

You will find that you will soon be able to ascertain the TP before the client tells you that you are on it. It is vital that your pressure begin lightly and gradually increase (up to 20 or 30 pounds or 9-14 kg of pressure) so that the client has a good chance of tolerating the pressure. If you begin with too much pressure, the client will likely experience too much pain to remain relaxed.

The cycle of pressure and then release will usually need to be repeated. Some TPs seem to deactivate readily and others require a number of attempts. The deactivation process probably correlates with the length of time the TP has been present

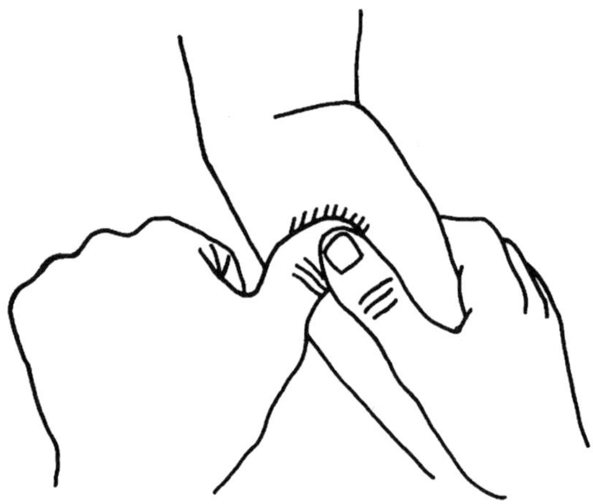

Figure 34. **Ischemic Compression Technique**

Place finger or thumb directly over trigger point and gradually apply direct pressure up to the client's level of tolerance.

and how soon it is precipitated again. Anecdotally, ischemic compression has been the most successful tool for managing the tender and trigger points of FS, in this author's experience.

Travell and Rinzler (1952) also suggest applying heavy pressure and spraying the trigger points. They said in 1952 that "The pain cycle is often terminated permanently by local block procedures with only transitory pharmacologic actions: procaine infiltration or dry needling of trigger areas, sustained heavy pressure on them, and spraying the overlying skin with ethyl chloride." (Fluoromethane has replaced ethyl chloride.)

In a study by Hong and colleagues (1993) comparing several physical therapy modalities, it was concluded that deep pressure soft tissue massage was more effective than thermotherapy or stretch and spray. This deep pressure massage was applied over a period of 10 to 15 minutes per treatment. This technique appears to be the same as ischemic compression except that in Hong's method stretching of the muscle fibers by the therapist's fingers occurs while the pressure is being applied, rather than placing muscle on a stretch prior to applying pressure.

After a few treatments, ischemic compression can readily be taught to another person so that it can be included in the home program. Either the helper can come to therapy with the client and learn the technique or the client can teach the helper simply by providing verbal guidance. It is most effective if performed often, perhaps 3 to 6 times per day, for well-established trigger points. No client can be seen in a clinic that often; therefore, someone who is with the client a lot is the ideal administrator of ischemic compression.

In fact, the client can usually apply ischemic compression on many areas independently on a daily basis. Some trigger points are within reach so the client can apply the technique in those areas. The client can also use a tennis ball to closely mimic

the technique by lying down on the ball and moving
the body to bring the tender/trigger point over the
ball. Body weight causes the ball to apply the compression. If the tennis ball is too rigid and causes
too much pain, a softer ball may be used. If a tennis
ball is not rigid enough, suggest a golf ball.

Some clients resist getting down on the floor. They
can utilize the same concept by placing the ball
between a wall and the body. If the ball drops to
the floor too often, the client can put the ball into
a long sock and hold one end of the sock. That way
the ball cannot drop and roll away.

Some clients lack sufficient strength in their fingers to apply the needed pressure to the tender/
trigger point. In this case, the ball in the sock is
really handy. For instance, if the tender point is in
the upper trapezius, the client can place the ball
over the trigger point and hold onto each end of the
sock. Then the client can apply pressure by pulling
the ends of the sock downward (see figure 35).

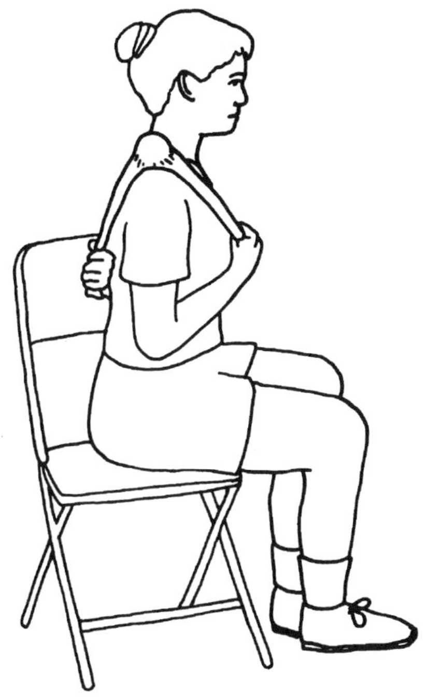

Figure 35. **Ischemic Compression**

A few words of warning are appropriate here.

1. Applying this compression increases pain for the duration of the compression.
   However, the client often remarks that it is "a good hurt." Often the compression will reproduce the client's symptoms and that might alarm the client or
   you initially. The technique will not cause damage (there should not be any
   bruising) so you can suggest that the client follow through for 3 to 4 days (5 to
   6 times per day) and then assess the results. Generally, the client will find that
   the trigger point is becoming less tender to the pressure and that the pain
   associated with that trigger point is slowly decreasing, if not gone entirely.

2. Remember that there are some people with FS who can hardly tolerate the
   weight of their clothing, so they will certainly not tolerate your compression.
   Encourage these people to work on desensitizing their trigger points at home
   so that they can begin to make use of this very effective tool. They should
   begin by gently rubbing the areas they can reach. Another way for the client
   to begin to build some tolerance to pressure is to use the stretch and spray tool
   for a while.

3. Begin gently. Listen to your client for cues telling you to increase or decrease
   pressure. Try to incorporate the muscle fiber stretching during the compression, as described by Hong and colleagues (1993).

4. The amount of pressure tolerated will vary from trigger point to trigger point
   in the same person.

5. As progress is made, the frequency of using the tool will decrease.

Breathing Exercise

Many breathing (relaxation) techniques can be beneficial for the person with FS. Use one that you know well and that the client can easily incorporate into daily routines. A simple one is a rhythmic breathing technique in which the client inhales for a count of 6 and holds the air in for a count of 3, then exhales for a count of 6 and holds the air out for a count of 3. If this is very easy for the client, suggest using the count of 8 and 4. Then progress to 10 and 5. You see the pattern: the holds are half the count of the inhalations and exhalations. Have the client continue this progression. The signal that determines the count to use is a slight feeling of stretching in the chest with full inhalation. Such an exercise will be of great benefit to those who have begun to breathe shorter and shorter due to anxiety, pain, or deconditioning by increasing awareness and relaxation. Often the pattern of upper chest breathing begins secondary to poor posture in which the abdominal muscles are weakened and rarely recruited, the diaphragm has lowered due to lack of support, and the thorax is kyphotic. This elicits greater than normal effort from the scalenes, which can precipitate trigger points in the scalenes (Zacharkow 1994).

Aerobic Exercise

As soon as possible, the client needs to begin some form of aerobic exercise 5 to 6 times per week. This does not mean that the client should join an aerobic dance class. Such an activity would likely be another example of "too much, too soon." There are a number of good options for aerobic work. The most accessible and least expensive for the largest number of people is walking. Swimming is a possibility, but most people with FS need a warm-water pool. Biking seems to work best with a stationary bike so that the client is not obliged to assume the forward bent position to reach the handle bars. With a stationary bike, the client can even sit upright and ignore the handlebars. Some clients have enjoyed using cross- country ski machines, treadmills, or stair machines to achieve their aerobic workouts.

Besides the systemic cardiovascular benefits that an increase in oxygenation provides, aerobic exercise can also develop more capillaries in the skeletal muscles. This development would make subsequent oxygenation of the muscle fibers more efficient by decreasing the distance that oxygen has to diffuse between the capillaries and muscle fibers (Klug, McAuley, and Clark 1989). Another beneficial change that aerobic work affects is increased myoglobin concentration, which also assists the diffusion of the oxygen within the muscle cell.

The client should assume the responsibility for doing this aerobic component of the program at home. You will need to guide the client with regard to intensity level, frequency, and duration of the workout. Remember to start lightly. Refer to the research section regarding the study in which it was found that people with FS could perform low-intensity endurance training without causing an exacerbation of symptoms (page 26). Their heart rate never exceeded 150 beats/minute (Mengshoel and Førre 1993). It is also helpful to refer to the formula for achieving an adequate training index of 42 each week (refer to American College of Sports

Medicine 1990). An adequate training index of 42 can be successfully achieved by increasing the frequency and/or the duration of exercise when the intensity must be kept low (Hagberg 1986). (This lower-intensity approach agrees with what is advised for the client with mitral valve prolapse also.) Advise your client that it might take as long as six months to become aerobically fit. The client should begin with only a few minutes of aerobic work at each session. Your client might be able to increase the duration by only one minute per session in a week's time. That's fine. Encourage the client to keep increasing the duration at this rate until able to attain the training index of 42. This achievement requires a lot of determination and encouragement to stick with the program.

There may be some starts and stops with getting this activity established as a regular part of the client's life. Your client probably already feels overwhelmed by everyday activities and will need encouragement in fitting this new one into her schedule. Also bear in mind that a regular exercise program is an especially difficult step for these clients if fatigue is a major complaint. Some people with FS experience overwhelming fatigue. To give us some perspective, Dr. Stuart Silverman of Los Angeles has said that "The fatigue of a 45-year-old woman with FS is approximately twice the fatigue of a 67-year-old patient with rheumatoid arthritis" (Silverman 1994).

Warm-Water Exercise

Many people with FS find that a warm pool provides them with the friendliest environment in which to exercise and that they feel better longer after a session in the warm water. Almost universally, people with FS do not like to be in cold water. This preference drastically limits the availability of an exercise pool as there are far more cold-water than warm-water pools. Water fitness educator Mary Essert (1994) says, "The buoyancy provided by the water prevents jolt to an already overwhelmed musculoskeletal system. For example, when standing neck deep in water, one experiences only one-tenth of one's body weight." She also points to the benefits of the hydrostatic pressure on swelling and on chest expansion for effective breathing. She suggests a pool with a temperature between 83 and 90 degrees. For aerobic work, the temperature should be under 88 degrees. Her guidelines include a warm-up consisting of water walking or water jogging, use of stretching and resistive work, and then a cool down using breathing and relaxation techniques. She emphasizes that people with FS need to work at a pace that is comfortable for them. If a warm-water pool is available for your clients, you will find that water exercise is a gentle, useful tool for many of them as they increase their level of activity. Another very practical point is that water exercise is "more cost efficient for patients with fibromyalgia because patients can do more sooner in the water" (Reichley 1995).

After you have initiated the portions of Stage 1 of the protocol that you deem useful, give the client 7 to 10 days to work on these tools. Then have the client return so that you can review everything up to this point, answer any questions the client has, and teach new tools from Stage 2.

STAGE 2

In this stage you will:

- teach light exercise and progress gradually
- continue soft tissue work and modalities as needed
- teach proper body mechanics
- help modify the client's work station

Scope

Remind the client that your goal is to teach tools for increasing functionality and managing pain and to have the client be able to use these tools independently. Schedule appointments with your client about 7 to 10 days apart.

You might find it helpful to develop a weekly chart for the client to help with keeping up the program you have devised together. The chart might include spaces for indicating the amount of aerobic exercise, stretches, and strengthening work to be done at regular intervals throughout each week.

Begin Stage 2 by reviewing what you have taught the client so far and answer any questions the client has. Reiterate important points, such as, be subtle, don't overdo the exercises, and be patient with your body.

Continue any modality you deem necessary, remembering that the client probably will not have access to them perpetually.

Range-of-Motion Exercises

Begin gentle, active range-of-motion exercises. Some of the most often needed ones are illustrated below. Use your basic knowledge to determine which other exercises would be helpful. Very often these are used by the client first thing in the morning to help alleviate the morning stiffness and the desire to stay in bed.

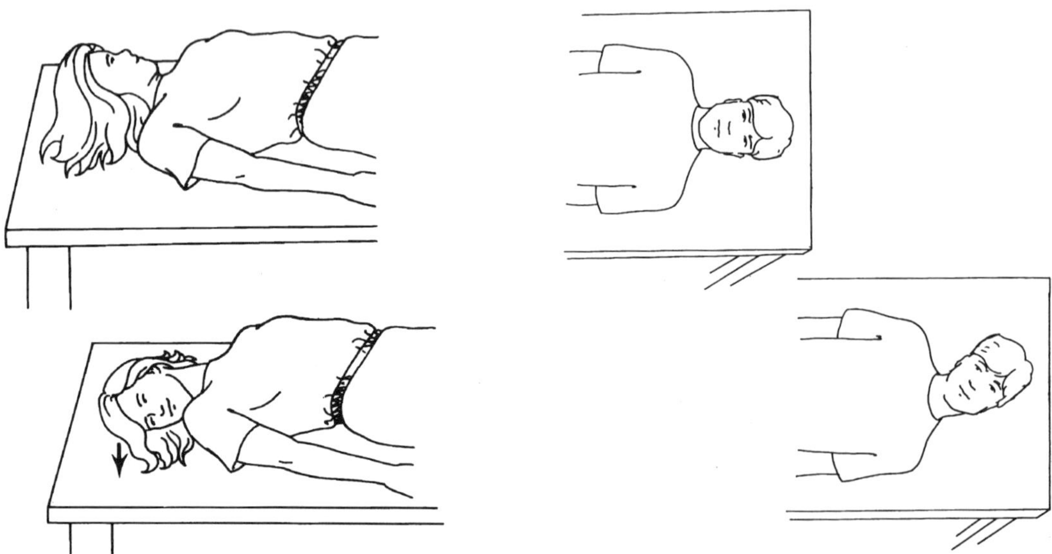

Figure 36. Cervical Range of Motion (Rotation)   *Figure 37.* Cervical Range of Motion (Sidebending)

By performing these exercises for active cervical range of motion in the supine position, gravity and postural tension are reduced and the client is able to move more freely. Instruct the client to move through the comfortable range and back to midline at a slow pace at first and then increase to a moderate pace.

Other exercises that are especially helpful in the morning are shown in the following pages. They are useful at other times during the day as well.

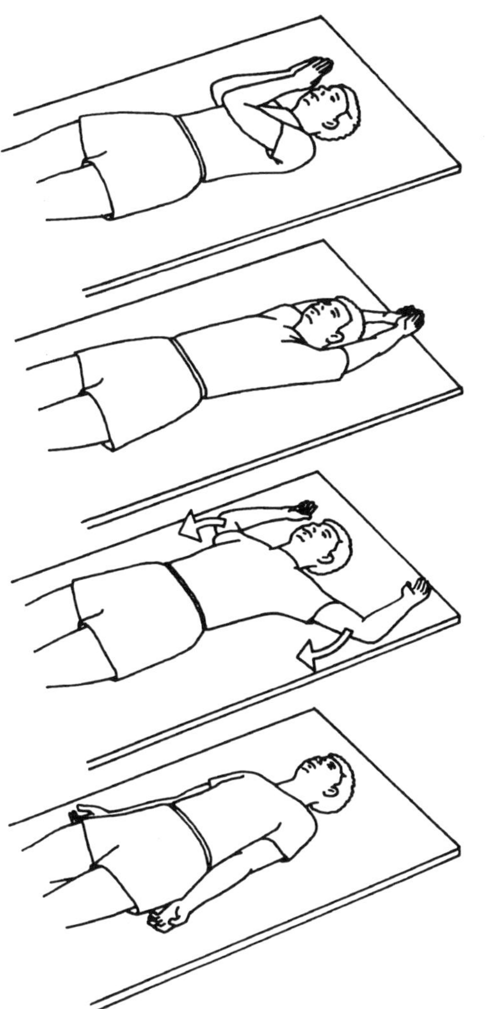

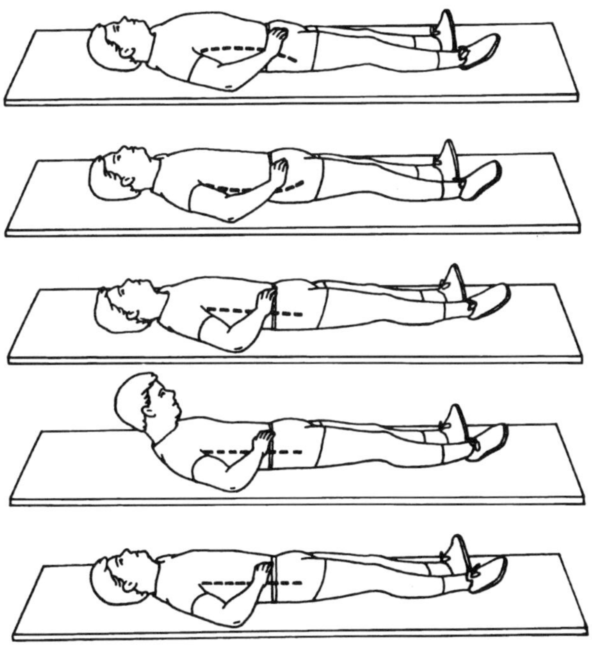

Figure 38. Scapula Retraction

Have the client lie on the back with the hands in the prayer position, then bring them up over the head. The client should squeeze the scapulae downward and toward each other as the forearms pronate. Have the client let the arms fall gently to the sides of the body. Teach this exercise in the upright position also.

Figure 39. Finding Neutral Spine

Have the client lie on the back and place the hands on the sides of the abdomen. Prompt the client to arch and flatten the back several times and feel the motion of the pelvis with the hands. Help the client find the mid-position (this is usually a pain-free spot) and maintain it. This is the neutral spine position. Encourage the client to incorporate this position into standing and sitting postures.

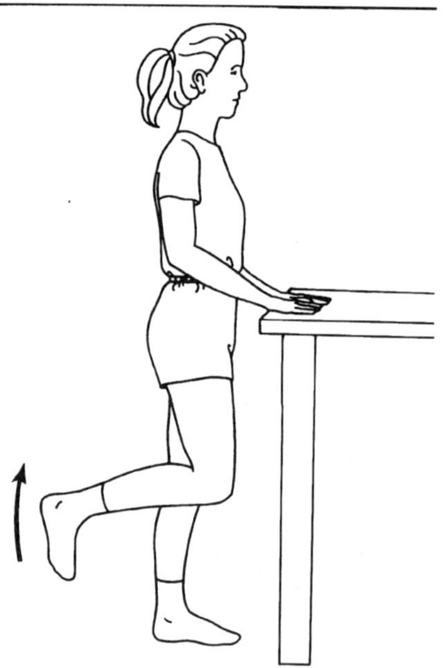

Figure 40. Standing Knee Flexion for Hamstring Strengthening

Have the client keep the spine neutral and bend first one knee, then the other. Later, resistance can be added.

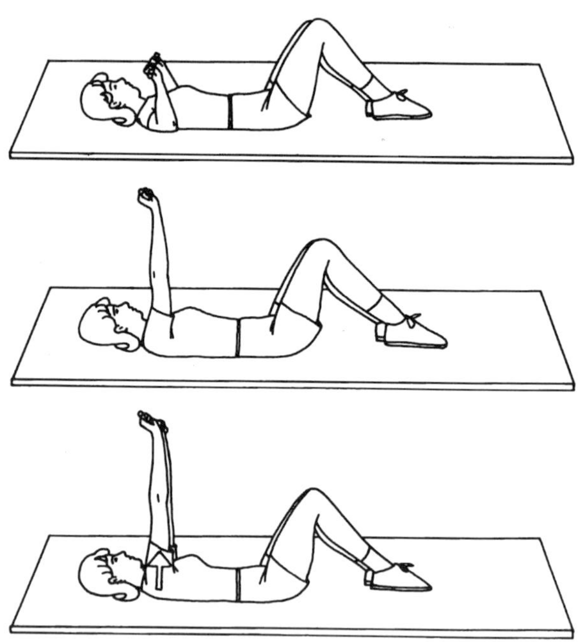

Figure 41. Scapular Protraction

Ask the client to lie on the back holding a bar (or nothing) with elbows bent. Have the client raise the bar while straightening the elbows. The bar should be pushed up high enough so that the shoulders raise off the bed toward the ceiling. Later, weights can be added to the bar. This exercise can also be done one arm at a time.

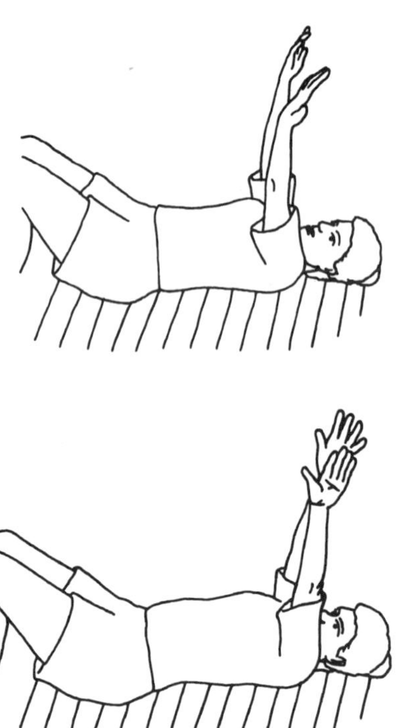

Figure 42. Active Shoulder Rotation

Have the client do this exercise slowly and completely in each direction. Ask the client if both shoulders feel the same during this range of motion exercise. Have your client strive to achieve symmetry with the shoulder rotations.

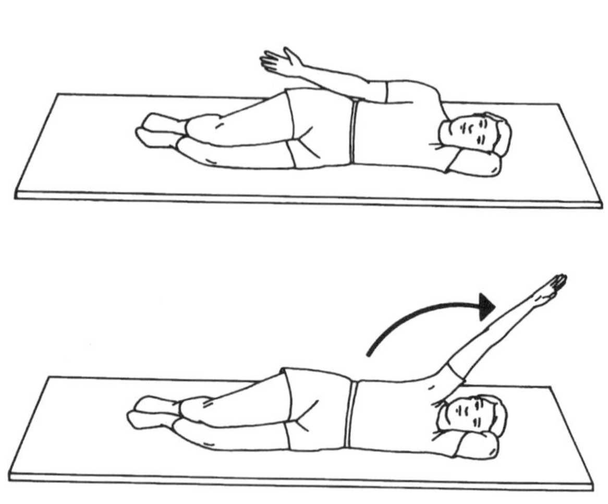

Figure 43. Sidelying Shoulder Abduction

Have the client lie on one side and raise the top arm overhead with elbow straight and thumb up. Then change sides and exercise the other arm. Resistance can be added later, in a very gradual manner.

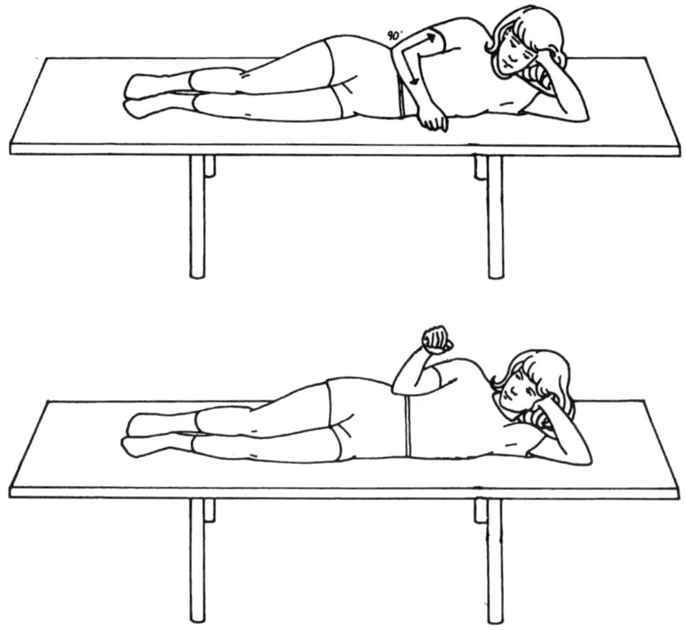

Figure 44. Sidelying Shoulder External Rotation

Have the client lie on one side and bend the top arm so that the elbow is resting on the waist. The arm should be bent at a 90-degree angle. Then prompt the client to raise the forearm and hand. Resistance can be added gradually.

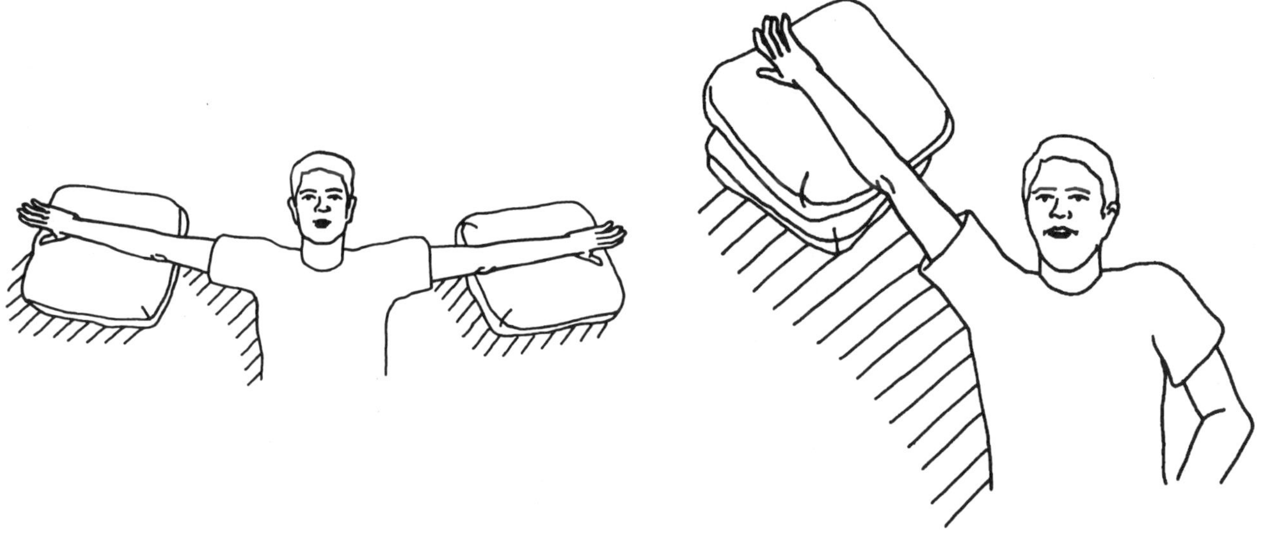

Figure 45. Supine Middle Trapezius Exercise

Have the client lie on the back with arms to the sides and push down into the pillows with the arms rolled into external rotation.

Figure 46. Supine Lower Trapezius Exercise

Have the client push down into the pillow with the shoulder in external rotation as shown. Advance the exercise by eliminating a pillow.

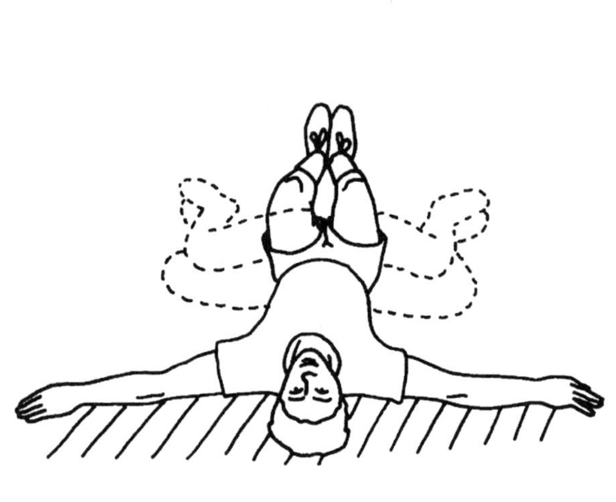

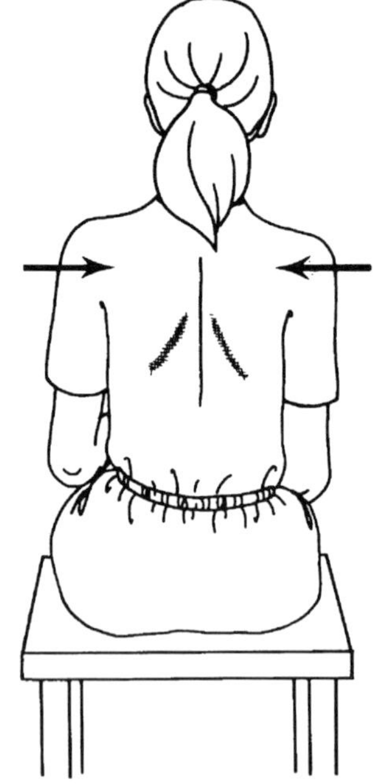

Figure 48. **Seated Scapula Setting**

While seated, the client should pull the scapulae downward and toward each other. Remind the client to always set the scapulae in this manner before picking up an object no matter how light or heavy.

Figure 47. **Trunk Rotation**

The client should bring the knees to the chest and rotate them slowly from side to side.

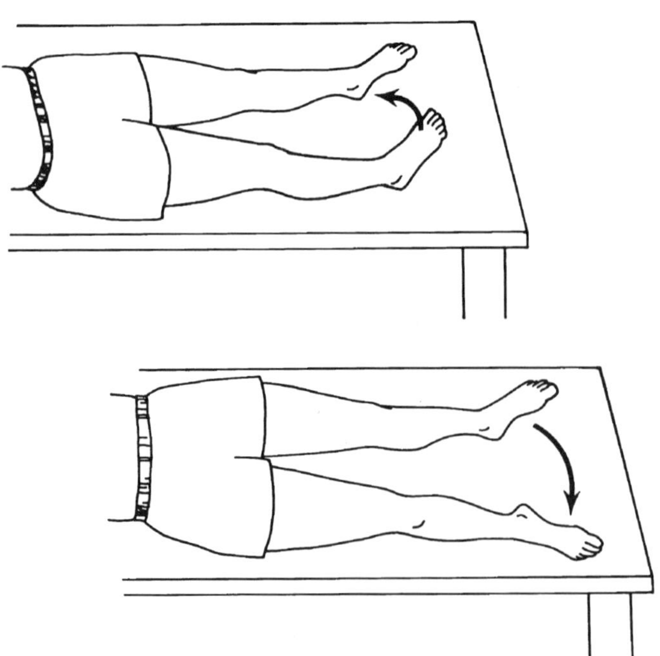

Figure 49. **Supine Hip Rotation**

Have the client lie supine and keep the legs out straight. Then prompt the client to slowly roll the legs so that the feet turn in and out as far as possible.

Body Mechanics

Continue with Stage 2 by instructing the client in safe body mechanics regarding lifting, pushing and pulling, and bending. Use visual aids, such as videos or printed material, as much as possible. Remember that you are a visual aid and your demonstration of proper body mechanics is very important. Then have the client practice the techniques for you so you can be sure the client understands and is able to use the information correctly. A few examples of safe body mechanics follow.

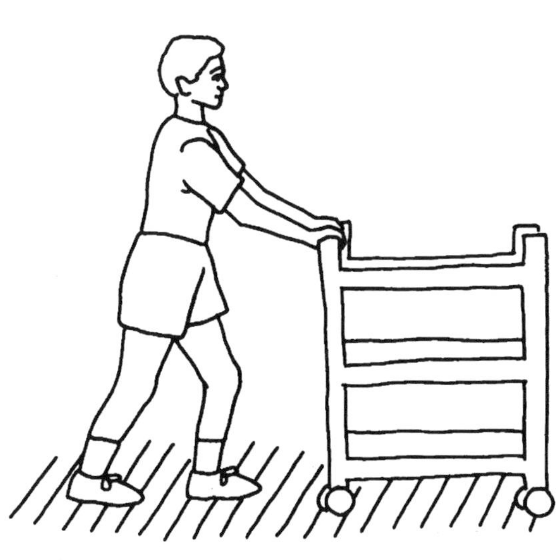

Figure 50. Pushing a Heavy Load

Teach the client that pushing is safer than pulling a heavy load. Remind the client to maintain neutral spine.

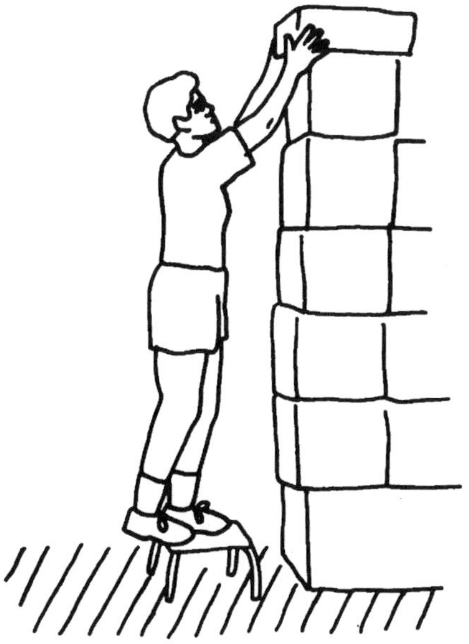

Figure 51. Reaching Overhead

Encourage the client to use a step stool when reaching overhead. Remind the client to maintain neutral spine.

Work Site Modification

Help your client apply the lessons in body mechanics to the workplace. Resume your conversation regarding the client's work situation that you began during the initial evaluation. If the client sits most of the day, offer the suggestions on page 90. If the client stands a lot during the day, the guidelines on page 92 are appropriate.

Advice for People Who Sit

Maintaining a neutral spine, or "keeping the spine in line," is the goal for people who sit a lot. To do so, keep your ears, shoulders, and hips aligned so that a straight line could be drawn between them. Try to avoid the C-curve-type sitting posture. Here are some tips to help you maintain a healthy back.

Sitting

Chair

- The height of the chair should be adjusted so that your feet are flat on the floor and your knees are at a level even with or slightly higher than your hips. Use a footstool if necessary. Sit with your rear to the rear of the chair.
- Use a chair with arms. The chair arms should be positioned directly under your shoulders. They should be at such a height that your forearms rest easily, elbows bent at about a right angle.
- Slide your chair under your desk as close to the work surface as you can. Bring your work to this work space in order to avoid twisting and reaching.

Desk: The height of the desk should be about even with your waist when you are seated.

Lumbar support: Use either a homemade rolled towel (customized to your size) or a commercial lumbar roll to place in the small of your back.

Keyboarding

- Instead of laying your work materials flat on the desk, use a rack or a clip to position them vertically.
- Place a wrist support in front of your keyboard. Make sure your screen is at eye level and is straight ahead of your body so that you do not need to twist to face it.

Reading: Hold reading materials vertically, rather than laying them flat on your work surface, and place your elbows on the desk. This posture will support your upper back, prevent slouching, and keep your head in line with your spine. (It is ideal to be seated in a high-back chair while reading.)

Deep breathing: Take several deep, cleansing breaths frequently.

Moving in Your Chair

Bending: Slide to the edge of your chair. Support your back with one hand on the desk and one foot in front of you. Then reach to pick up an object from the floor.

Standing up: Slide to the edge of your chair. Place one foot forward and one foot under the chair. Keep your back in the neutral position and use your leg muscles to push you up. Do get up and move around often to relieve pressure on the low back.

Turning: Keep feet and hips pointed in the same direction as you turn. Move your body as a single unit and avoid twisting.

Phoning: Never hold the receiver between your head and shoulder. If you do, attach a support to the receiver to soften the angle between your head and shoulder. Ideally, use a head set. Otherwise, switch the receiver from side to side frequently.

Exercising: Do appropriate exercises regularly at your desk. Use those that you have been taught by your therapist.

Driving

Seat position: Move the car seat forward far enough to allow easy access to pedals without having to reach for them. This position should allow your knees to be level with your hips. Slide your rear to the rear of the seat. Use a lumbar support or place a small wedge under your rear, high side toward the back of the seat.

Posture: Sit straight with both hands on the wheel. Use your head support by making sure it is high enough so that the back of your head can rest on it. To avoid tension buildup, use armrests if available.

Adapted with permission from: SportsMed Orthopaedics and Rehabilitation (Wheaton Orthopaedics, Ltd.) Carol Stream, IL.

Advice for People Who Stand and Lift

Standing

Use a step stool or book: Stand with one foot supported on a step stool or book. Anything available may be used to elevate the foot. Change feet often to relieve pressure on the lower back and decrease the lower-back curve. If possible, sit down periodically.

Practice good posture: Ears, shoulders, hips, knees, and ankles should be in good alignment so that a straight line can be drawn through these points. Think of a string attached to the crown of your head. If that string is pulled upward, your body will assume good neutral alignment.

Wear comfortable, low-heeled shoes: Select shoes that offer good support in the arch and a firm heel counter.

Use opposite motions: Perform motions and assume positions that are opposite to the ones that you use all day. In other words, if you bend forward most of the day, take short breaks and bend backward.

Lifting

Back bending: Prior to heavy lifting, or in between repetitive lifting, place your hands on the small of the back and bend backward gently several times.

Correct lifting technique:

- Plan ahead by clearing your pathway and minimizing the distance you must carry the object.
- Get as close to the object as possible and use a firm footing with a wide, staggered stance.
- Maintain neutral alignment in your back and use your legs to lower your body. Keep the abdominals tightened.
- Keep the object close to your body.
- Use your leg and buttock muscles to lift the load, keeping your back in neutral alignment.
- **After** you are upright, shift your feet in order to turn your body. Turning while lifting places excess stress on the back.

Exercise: Do exercises for lower-back conditioning to keep the back supporting muscles strong and flexible.

Adapted with permission from: SportsMed Orthopaedics and Rehabilitation (Wheaton Orthopaedics, Ltd.) Carol Stream, IL.

Upgraded Exercises

Begin to progress your client's exercise program slowly. Use your knowledge and understanding of your client to determine which exercises should come next. Remember that the following exercises are only examples. There are many possibilities.

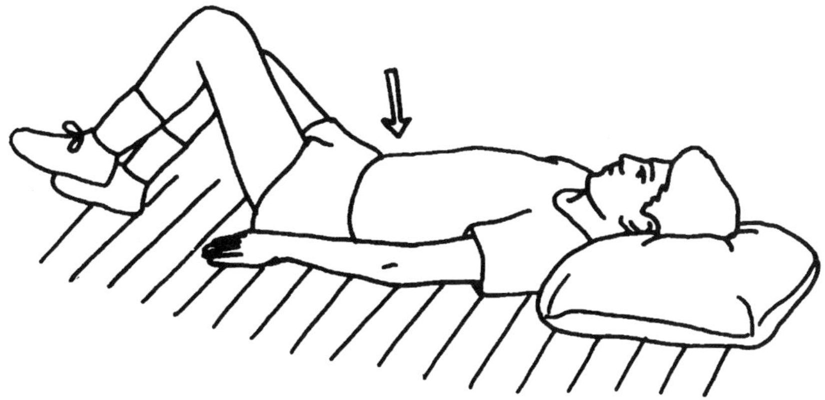

***Figure 52.* Neutral Spine with Stepping**

Have the client lie supine and tighten the abdominal muscles to find neutral spine (pelvic tilt). The client should maintain the neutral spine while lifting one knee and then setting the foot back down. Relax. Repeat the process using the other leg. Be sure the client maintains neutral spine until both feet are on the floor. (A good idea for upgrading the exercises is to continue with the neutral spine program.)

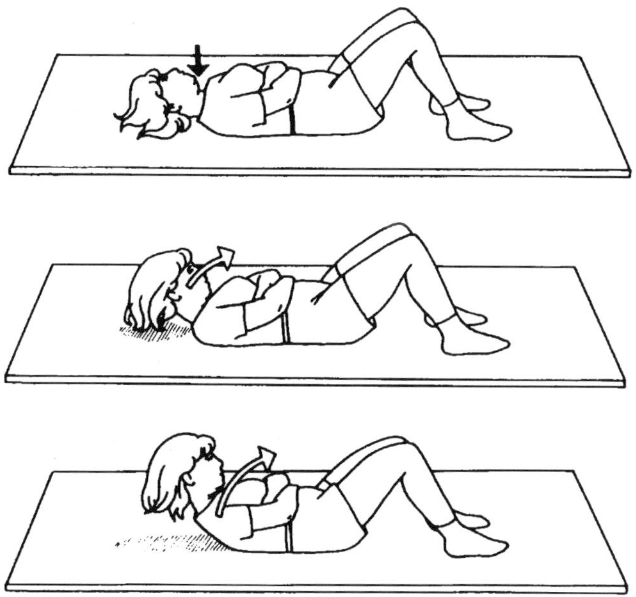

***Figure 53.* Partial Curl-Up**

Ask the client to lie on the back with knees bent and raise the head, shoulders, and shoulder blades off the floor. Then return to start position. Caution the client to do these exercises slowly.

Scope

By this stage, your client is well on the way to being independent in using the treatment program and the tools available. In Stage 3 you will finalize the program and discharge the client. Remember that you cannot expect the patient to be 100% better than at the beginning of therapy. However, by this point there will usually be some nice improvement and both of you will have a positive feeling about going in the right direction.

Review and Upgrade Exercises

Review and upgrade the client's exercise program. At this point, the client is probably ready to begin some light resistive work using small free weights (or items from the pantry), light tubing, or tension bands. These programs are second nature to you as a therapist. Choose the ones that your client needs the most but remember to start with lighter weights and fewer repetitions than you do with other clients. When it is time to increase the load, do so very gradually. This type of training is important for the skeletal muscles for lots of reasons. One particularly interesting reason involves the changes that occur only in the muscles that are actually used in training. For example, "the activity of the mitochondrial marker enzyme succinate dehydrogenase was significantly elevated in the trained leg when compared to the activity in the contralateral, untrained leg" in subjects who rode a stationary bicycle with one leg (Klug, McAuley, and Clark 1989). Also, the muscle metabolism shifted to utilization of fats in the trained leg. Therefore, these researchers suggest carefully selecting exercises for clients with FS in order to facilitate these potential changes in the affected muscles.

Beyond the exercises you choose for your client, some of the most typical exercises that people with FS need target the scapula stabilizers. Some suggestions have been offered in Stage 2. The following are suggestions for more advanced work.

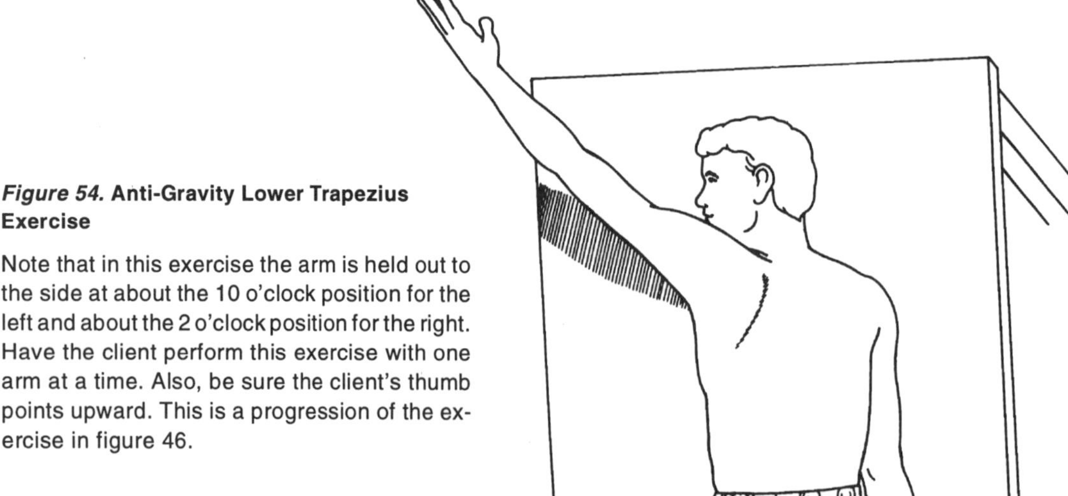

Figure 54. Anti-Gravity Lower Trapezius Exercise

Note that in this exercise the arm is held out to the side at about the 10 o'clock position for the left and about the 2 o'clock position for the right. Have the client perform this exercise with one arm at a time. Also, be sure the client's thumb points upward. This is a progression of the exercise in figure 46.

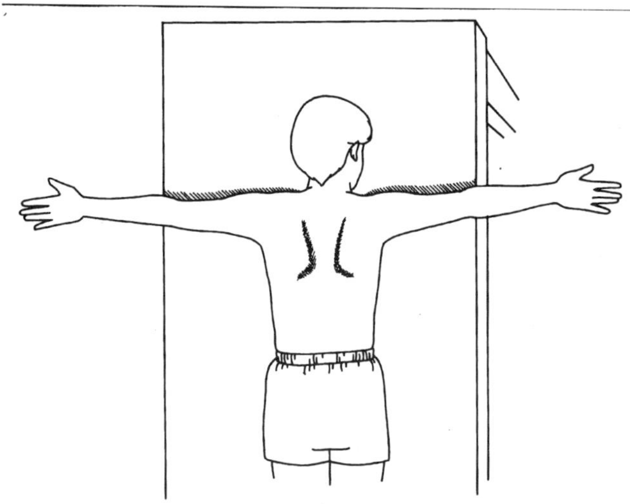

Figure 55. Anti-Gravity Middle Trapezius Exercise

Have the client raise the arms together, symmetrically. Be sure that the client does not raise the upper body. Small weights can eventually be added to the client's hands or more proximal points along the arms. Instruct the client to turn the thumbs up. This is a progression of the exercise in figure 45.

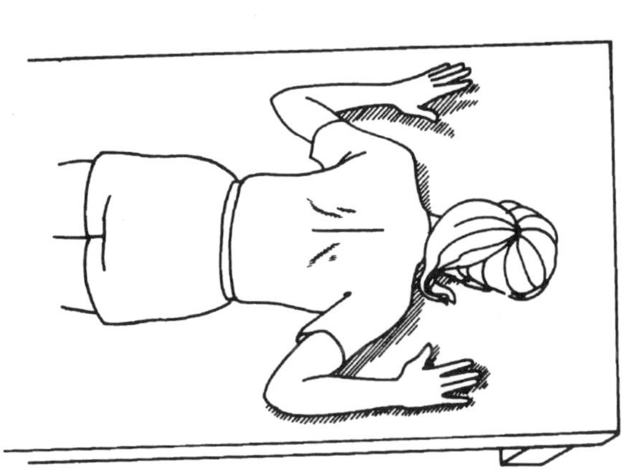

Figure 56. Scapula Retraction

Have the client lie on the stomach with the elbows bent at the sides of the body. Prompt the client to raise the forearms while keeping the head still.

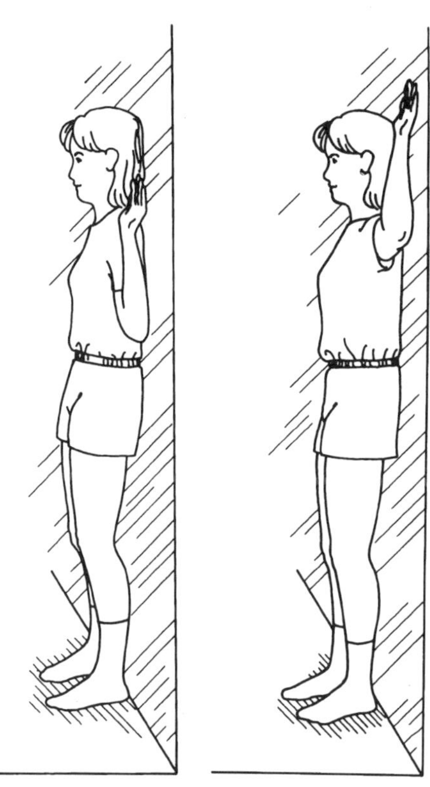

Figure 57. Scapula Retraction with Shoulder Elevation

Have the client stand with the back flattened against a wall. Remind the client to tighten abdominal muscles and start the exercise with the arms in the position shown in the illustration. Have the client raise the arms along the wall until the back can no longer be kept flat against the wall. Relax. Repeat.

Reassure and Congratulate

In this stage, remember to reassure the client and offer congratulations on the hard work put forth. Depending on the client's tolerance, continue to upgrade the exercise program and utilize fitness center equipment if the client will have access to that type of equipment. Always emphasize the high-repetition, low-load approach to weight lifting or use of exercise machines. Be sure to make use of circuit training also.

By this time, the client has learned the following tools: stretching, aerobic exercise, soft tissue mobilization techniques, breathing techniques, moist heat, stretch and spray, posture modification, proper body mechanics, work-site modification, and strengthening exercises.

Release Client from Formal Therapy

The effectiveness of each tool will vary from client to client as well as from day to day for the same client. It is important that the client understand all of the tools and have ownership of them in order to utilize them to the greatest benefit. Upon achieving that understanding, the client will be ready to be released from formal therapy. Try to make yourself accessible (by phone at least) to answer any questions that may arise. Usually, by this point most clients have become very knowledgeable and really do not need to rely on you anymore. Occasionally, clients need short-term help at some point after they have been discharged if too many precipitating factors occur within a short period of time and the client becomes overwhelmed. A few treatments with you will help the client to regain control. For the most part, clients with FS readily accept the responsibility of self-management and are successful with it once they are equipped with the proper tools.

Jobs and Disability

How does FS affect people in their occupations? How do chosen occupations affect people with FS? In a recent study of people with FS and their occupations reported by Waylonis, Ronan, and Gordon (1994), a group of 321 people with FS were surveyed to ascertain which kinds of jobs aggravate the symptoms. They found that 20% of the group worked in general office settings, 14% worked in health-related areas, 11% worked in education, 8% were unemployed, and 7% worked in retail positions. The major aggravating activities reported were: typing (37%), prolonged sitting (37%), prolonged standing and walking (27%), stress (21%), heavy lifting or bending (19%), repetitive moving and lifting (18%), prolonged writing (9%), maintaining arms in an unsupported position (8%), prolonged telephone use (8%), and environmental discomfort (8%). The researchers point out that some occupations were not represented among the survey respondents, yet clients working in jobs other than those listed above are often seen in their clinic. An example of one such job is assembly line work. These researchers suggest that job task rotation during a work shift be instituted for people with FS because a protracted period of time at a single task seems to increase symptoms. It is expected that this type of accommodation will help to reduce the number of work days lost.

Some people with FS have difficulty continuing to perform their jobs. Of those in this group, some apply for disability pensions or change their jobs. According to a 1992 survey reported in a recent newsletter, "11% of patients were receiving disability pensions, 33% said that they had to change jobs because of FS and 54% were having difficulties with routine daily living activities" (AFSA Update 1994). As noted by Dr. Wolfe (1994), the operant social system has a major influence on work disability designations. Therefore, 24% of the Swedish FS patients were receiving disability pensions as opposed to 6% to 8% of American FS patients. He also reported on several other studies that demonstrated 30% of people with FS in the United States had changed jobs because of FS.

The term *disability* needs definition. According to Dr. Wolfe (1993a), when discussing a person's ability to engage in a job, the term should be referred to as *work disability*. He recommends this term because a person can be quite disabled functionally but still not be work disabled. Dr. Wolfe details the process physicians are required to complete on the person's behalf in trying to satisfy the lawyers and insurance companies when a person has applied for a disability pension. He also discusses the difficulty in determining the etiology of FS but concludes that in some cases a reasonable connection can be made between an injury and the onset of FS. He offers guidance on the process of justifying work disability awards but points out that "All of us are best off if we can work in productive capacities, particularly the individual with fibromyalgia. But this may take job change and additional education" (Wolfe 1993a).

These statistics should stimulate our thinking about ways to modify job sites and job tasks where feasible in order to help keep people with FS functioning and able to perform their jobs. If that is not feasible and a change is necessary, then some counseling and thoughtful consideration regarding the new job requirements is in order. In cases in which people with FS have actually quit working altogether, significant pain relief has not generally been achieved.

Other Professionals Involved in Care

Because so many aspects of a person are affected by FS, one might expect to see several different health professionals involved in care. This is, in fact, true and has sometimes been carried to the extreme, taking a large financial and emotional toll. Centralizing the professional care would certainly be beneficial. To this end, more and more multifaceted programs for the treatment of FS are being developed and they seem to be producing good results for the clients. One such program in Oregon provides a good model and utilizes patient education, myofascial therapy, physical conditioning, sleep quality improvement, and psychological counseling (Bennett et al. 1991). This program is augmented by a monthly support group that is conducted by a nurse-educator or a psychologist.

A physician who understands FS and its management should be at the helm of the health-care team. Beyond an accurate diagnosis, the physician will typically monitor the client's medications, possibly offer TrP injections, sympathetic blocks, or dry needling of the TrPs, provide reassurance and information, and refer the client to other appropriate health-care professionals.

A psychologist or psychiatrist who understands chronic pain and FS and the toll they take on a person's energy and joy can be invaluable in the client's progress. Coping strategies, such as cognitive restructuring, visualization, biofeedback, and relaxation, can be wonderful additions to a person's repertoire of tools.

A massage therapist who understands FS can also assist the client with relaxation and specific tender/trigger point release, thus providing much-needed relief from pain and assistance in enhancing functional abilities. An occupational therapist can help with modifying work stations, devising any splinting necessary, and guiding exercises.

A nutritionist who is knowledgeable about FS, irritable bowel syndrome, and the relationship of oxidative stress and chronic problems can be of great assistance in helping the client with FS to manage some of the symptoms.

How to Start a Support Group

Because participation in a self-help group can be so important for people with FS and because there are not enough groups available, this section has been written to encourage you, as a caring therapist, to facilitate a new group in your area. There are many ways to initiate a new group as you will hear if you attend a seminar on FS and speak with other participants. Several books have been written about starting support groups. These resources can be found in your local library. Here is just one description of the start-up of one support group specifically for fibromyalgia. Perhaps this account of the start of the Fibromyalgia Association of DuPage County, Illinois, will encourage you to start a group in your community.

A physiatrist in our community, Dr. Frank Lagattuta, had hinted to me several times that "these people need a support group." But I didn't know how to start one and I certainly didn't have the time to do so. Or so I thought. In June of 1990, a co-worker and I attended the first national seminar on FS in Columbus, Ohio. Two important things happened there. One was that we met a massage therapist from our community, Mary Ann Phemister, R.N., who was very enthusiastic about our working together to form a support group. The other seminal event was hearing Dr. Ernesto Vasquez speak powerfully on the great good that could be shared with a lot of people through the vehicle of a support group.

When we returned after the seminar, we had a lunch meeting with our physiatrist friend. We were all convinced that a support group was something that needed to happen and that we would give it an honest try, even though none of us were knowledgeable about the mechanics of the task. We agreed that education was the number one priority because once people stopped rejoicing over finally having received a diagnosis, they were frustrated at knowing very little about FS and were unable to explain it to friends and relatives. They also needed more information in order to be able to accept and cope with this mysterious syndrome. Since we had determined education to be our top priority, we recognized that we would need speakers and literature to help people understand FS. Brainstorming yielded a number of possibilities for speakers. We also gathered articles on FS and copies of the *Fibromyalgia Network* newsletter, as well as videos of the Columbus seminar, and made those available.

Our other main priority was to provide support for those who suffer from FS and their families. We decided to divide the meetings into two parts. One part would be dedicated to education and the other to sharing and supporting.

The next items that needed to be considered were location and publicity. The waiting room at our clinic provided the answer to one problem. As a public service, local newspapers published a notice of our first meeting in their community calendars. We also envisioned a newsletter as a way to communicate with those interested in the group.

Since we wanted to serve refreshments and some speakers request an honorarium, we realized that we would need to charge a small fee to participants in order to cover these costs. We decided that we would not charge the family members who came to provide support.

On a wing and a prayer, we held our first meeting two months after attending the seminar in Columbus. So many people attended that our room was immediately too small and we began looking for a new space. Since that first meeting, we have met in the public library's community room, a bank's community room, the cafeteria of a hospital, and now, five years later, we are meeting at a convention/resort center at no charge. You never know what facilities are available until you ask.

What has transpired in our group since the beginning? We have heard from many speakers, including several physiatrists, a rheumatologist, a psychologist, a warm-water exercise expert, a massage therapist, a nutritionist, a dentist, a rehab nurse, a chiropractor, and, of course, a physical therapist. We learned to break into small groups for sharing time rather than try to do so with all 30 to 35 people at the meeting. We stopped serving refreshments because it became too messy and stressful. We started a lending library and we publish a newsletter that we now call *Fibromation*. We alternate education meetings with support meetings now rather than try to split each meeting into two parts. My role has shifted to phone support and the leadership of the group has shifted to the participants. In fact, one of these new leaders, B. J. Davis, organized and guided us through a weekend seminar a few years ago that was attended by people from throughout the state.

Since the inception of our group, there has been a lot of growth in number of participants, in understanding of each other and of ourselves, and in depth of experience. We know a lot more about how to start a support group now. (I recommend checking into your state laws regarding forming a not-for-profit organization early in the process.) The gratifying fact is that it happened, no matter how naively or timidly. You can make it happen in your community, too. Please do.

Some helpful resources:

Coping with Fibromyalgia
by Beth Ediger
This book is available from the
Fibromyalgia Association of
Central Ohio.

*Fibromyalgia: A Handbook for
Self-Care and Treatment*
by Janet A. Hulme, M.A., PT.
Published by:
Phoenix Publishing Company
P.O. Box 8231
Missoula, MT 59807

Fibromyalgia Network
P.O. Box 31750
Tucson, AZ 85751-1750
(520) 290-5508 (phone)
(520) 290-5550 (fax)

The Fibromyalgia Syndrome
by Mary Anne Saathoff, R.N., B.S.N.
You can obtain this book from the
Fibromyalgia Association of
Central Ohio.

When Muscle Pain Won't Go Away
by Gayle Backstrom
You can find this book in your local
bookstore or library.
Published by:
Taylor Publishing Company
1550 W. Mockingbird Lane
Dallas, TX 75235

Fibromyalgia Association of
Central Ohio
3545 Olentangy River Road
Columbus, Ohio 43214
(614) 262-2000

Fibromyalgia Association of
Greater Washington
P.O. Box 2373
Centreville, WA 22020
Send for their list of audio and video
tapes on fibromyalgia syndrome.

The Haworth Press, Inc.
10 Alice Street
Binghamton, NY 13904
Ask for information regarding the
Journal of Musculoskeletal Pain.

Also refer to page 60 for more suggestions.

■ Appendix

Case Studies

The following three case studies have been taken from medical charts and interviews with clients with FS. An attempt has been made to describe cases of varying intensity of symptomatology.

Case Study 1

A professional scientist was involved in a motor vehicle accident and within two months developed numbness of the left upper extremity into the lateral three fingers, prickliness in the lateral toes of the left foot, aching throughout the left side of the back and neck, sharp pain near the left scapula, and spasm activity in the left sternocleidomastoid muscle. At her initial evaluation in physical therapy, she rated her pain as 4 or 5 out of 10 (0 being no pain and 10 being intolerable pain). She felt that her left upper extremity was weaker than her right and she complained of not sleeping well. X-rays were negative. Her cervical range of motion was limited to 80% in forward flexion, 10% in extension, 50% in left rotation, 30% in right rotation, 30% in left sidebending, and 20% in right sidebending. In the lumbar area, all ranges were within normal limits except extension, which was 10% and painful. Multiple trigger points were noted along her occipital ridge, in the upper trapezius muscles, the infraspinatus muscles, levator muscles, lower trapezius muscles, and along the vertebral border of her scapulae. The tingling in the left fingers could be reproduced by ischemic compression of a trigger point in the left infraspinatus muscle.

She was treated with hot packs followed by soft tissue work emphasizing ischemic compression to the trigger points. She was instructed in using a tennis ball at home for this purpose. She also performed stretching exercises for upper trapezius and levator muscles. She utilized neck retraction, active cervical sidebending, and rotation in supine as well as shoulder elevation with her back against the wall.

Within four weeks, her cervical range of motion had improved to full flexion, 90% of rotation bilaterally, and 60% of sidebending bilaterally. She reported that the numbness in her left upper extremity had improved but was still present. She was sleeping better. The discomfort and the spasm in the sternocleidomastoid had improved. She noted that carrying luggage and reaching overhead in her lab aggravated her pain. At that time, light resistive exercises were added for shoulders and scapular retraction. She began low-level aerobic work also.

Three weeks later she was free from discomfort except for a little stiffness in the morning and after prolonged sitting. She felt that she was well enough to discontinue formal therapy. She had exercised on her own from the beginning of her therapy so her sessions were dedicated to soft tissue work and upgrading her exercise program.

Case Study 2

This young woman is a secretary and sought medical care originally because of soreness in her right forearm, which appeared to be an overuse syndrome of her wrist extensors secondary to uninterrupted hours of typing. Anti-inflammatory medications were tried as well as phonophoresis and soft tissue work to the lateral epicondyle area and to the muscle bellies of the extensor muscles. When she saw the physician five weeks later, she had obtained some relief of the forearm pain but was complaining of more generalized pain. Thorough testing failed to point to a specific diagnosis. She went away for vacation and felt fine until she returned to work where she had to sit in a cold draft and faced a heavy load of typing. This triggered another flare of her symptoms.

Initially she was treated for lateral epicondylitis in physical therapy but noted that the symptoms moved around. Further inspection revealed trigger points. The compression of a trigger point in the infraspinatus reproduced her forearm pain. She also mentioned that she had disturbed sleep. By the next session, it was noted that she was guarded in ambulation. Upon inquiry she said that she felt pain in her upper back, knee, and elbow. Her medication was changed to Indocin. Within three days she had such a severe headache she had to go to the emergency room for help. She attributed the headache to the Indocin. After lab work showed nothing, she was diagnosed with fibromyalgia. She was given an article about fibromyalgia and she agreed that it seemed to describe her situation. She also noted increases in her pain with weather changes and with increased stress.

Therapy consisted of various approaches that included microcurrent to the arms, phonophoresis to the epicondylitis, spray and stretch, gentle range-of-motion exercises, soft tissue mobilization, ischemic compression, hot packs, postural correction, low-level aerobic work, and general strengthening exercises. About two months into her therapy she was able to say that the exercises were becoming easier.

Her work site was eventually adjusted, which made a big difference for her. Of special importance was the addition of armrests to her typing chair. The height of her chair seat was also adjusted. She tried a wrist cock-up splint to relieve the stress on the wrist extensors at the elbow with some measure of success. Her job tasks were modified for a while so that she typed less and filed more. However, this led to increased pain in her upper back and soon low back pain ensued.

She joined a fitness center to better conduct her home exercise program. In therapy she was directed in how to upgrade her program. A lot of encouragement was given throughout her frustrating experience. She continued to work and was well supported there also. After six months of therapy, she felt she was ready to manage her case and was discharged. At a follow-up visit, she reported that her symptoms were 90% improved if she exercised regularly.

Case Study 3

Patient 3 underwent a discectomy on the right at L4-5. She had a good recovery and returned to her job as an attorney for a large company within three months. Soon she experienced a twisting and lifting incident which led to left lower extremity radiculopathy, numbness in the right foot, and pain in the left shoulder radiating down the arm.

Her internal medicine physician ran tests for rheumatoid arthritis, multiple sclerosis, and lupus, which were negative. An MRI did show an HNP at L5-S1. EMG confirmed the left L5 radiculopathy. During this period she was often unable to get up to go to the bathroom in the morning without her husband's assistance. Her arms also felt "dead" and she could not raise them. Multiple trigger points in the cervical and thoracic muscles and in her left lower lumbar area were noted within two months of the twisting incident. At that point she was diagnosed with fibromyalgia. She also remembers having anxiety attacks while driving that rendered her unable to continue to drive. She would have to pull off the road and wait until the attack subsided.

She began walking and swimming in addition to doing spinal stabilization exercises. She had to give up the swimming because the chlorine bothered her too much. She worked up to walking 2 to 3 miles per day and tried to move her arms vigorously during the walk. These exercises were helping, but not enough.

She had to quit her job, which was very stressful psychologically and financially. She needed to have a restriction on lifting as well as a limitation of 30 minutes of sitting at a time. Her commute to work alone caused exacerbation of symptoms. Therefore, she began to practice law out of her home on a part-time basis. In three years, she finally felt strong enough to open an office for her law practice.

As far as medications were concerned, she tried Elavil for a while but developed side effects that she could not tolerate, such as blurred vision and loss of coordination. She also used Tylenol 3 off and on but found that this contributed to headaches and constipation, which were not acceptable either. For a while she took magnesium. It helped with spasms and she did feel better generally.

She found that her best tools were exercise, especially walking or biking outside, using a heating pad, and relaxation techniques. She noted that exercising to the point of sweating made her feel the best. Massage had been a wonderful aid to relaxation but she could not continue that due to the cost.

Interestingly, she related that she has several first-degree relatives who suffer from major psychiatric problems.

References

Abraham, G. E., and J. D. Flechas. 1992. Management of fibromyalgia syndrome: Rationale for the use of magnesium and malic acid. *Journal of Nutritional Medicine* 3:49-59.

AFSA Update. May 1994. Getting to the point. *AFSA Update.* 1(1):1-2. Bakersfield, CA: The American Fibromyalgia Syndrome Association, Inc.

Ahles, T. A., S. A. Khan, M. B. Yunus, D. A. Spiegel, and A. T. Masi. 1991. Psychiatric states of patients with primary fibromyalgia, patients with rheumatoid arthritis, and subjects without pain: A blind comparison of DSM-III diagnoses. *American Journal of Psychiatry* 148:1721-1726.

Ahles, T. A., M. B. Yunus, and A. T. Masi. 1987. Is chronic pain a variant of depressive disease? The case of primary fibromyalgia syndrome. *Pain* 29:105-111.

Ahles, T. A., M. B. Yunus, S. D. Railey, J. M. Bradley, and A. T. Masi. 1984. Psychological factors associated with primary fibromyalgia syndrome. *Arthritis and Rheumatism* 27:1101-1106.

American College of Sports Medicine. 1990. The recommended quantity and quality of exercise for developing and maintaining cardiorespiratory and muscular fitness in healthy adults. *Medicine and Science in Sports and Exercise* 22:265-274.

Backman, E., A. Bengtsson, M. Bengtsson, C. Lennmarken, and K. G. Henriksson. 1988. Skeletal muscle function in primary fibromyalgia: Effect of regional sympathetic blockade with guanethidine. *Acta Neurologica Scandinavica* 77:187-191.

Bell, Iris. 1993. Medical neurobiology of CFS and FMS conference review, part II. *Fibromyalgia Network* 23(Oct.):12. Written and published by Kristin Thorson. Bakersfield, CA.

Bengtsson, A., and M. Bengtsson. 1988. Regional sympathetic blockade in fibromyalgia. *Pain* 33:161-7.

Bengtsson, A., K. G. Henriksson, and J. Larsson. 1986a. Reduced high-energy phosphate levels in the painful muscles of patients with primary fibromyalgia. *Arthritis and Rheumatism* 29:817-821.

Bengtsson, A., K. G. Henriksson, and J. Larsson. 1986b. Muscle biopsy in primary fibromyalgia. *Scandinavian Journal of Rheumatology* 15:1-6.

Bennett, R. M. 1990. Chronic fatigue syndrome: New insights in diagnosis and office management. *Modern Medicine* 58(3):50-62.

Bennett, R. 1993a. The origin of myopain: An integrated hypothesis of focal muscle changes and sleep disturbance in patients with the fibromyalgia syndrome. *Journal of Musculoskeletal Pain* 1(3/4):95-112.

Bennett, R. M. 1993b. NIH's scientific workshop on FMS paves direction for future research: Exercise. *Fibromyalgia Network* 22(July):7. Written and published by Kristin Thorson. Bakersfield, CA.

Bennett, R. M., S. Campbell, C. Burckhardt, S. Clark, C. O'Reilly, and A. Wiens. 1991. A multidisciplinary approach to fibromyalgia management. *Journal of Musculoskeletal Medicine* 8(11): 21-32.

Bennett, R. M., S. R. Clark, S. M. Campbell, and C. S. Burkhardt. 1992. Low levels of somatomedin-C in patients with the fibromyalgia syndrome: A possible link between sleep and muscle pain. *Arthritis and Rheumatism* 35:113-116.

Bennett, R. M., S. R. Clark, L. Goldberg, D. Nelson, R. D. Bonafede, J. Porter, and D. Specht. 1989. Aerobic fitness in the fibrositis syndrome: A controlled study of respiratory gas exchange and 133 xenon clearance from exercising muscle. *Arthritis and Rheumatism* 32:454-460.

Bennett, R. M., R. A. Gatter, S. M. Campbell, and R. P. Andrews. 1988. A comparison of cyclobenza-prine and placebo in the management of fibrositis: A double-blind controlled study. *Arthritis and Rheumatism* Dec. 31(12):1535-1542.

Bennett, R. M., H. A. Smythe, and F. Wolfe. 1992. Recognizing fibromyalgia. *Patient Care* March 15:211-228.

Boisset-Pioro, M. H., J. M. Esdaile, and M. A. Fitzcharles. 1995. Sexual and physical abuse in females with fibromyalgia syndrome. *Arthritis and Rheumatism* 38:235-241.

Buskila, D., D. D. Gladman, P. Longevitz, S. Urowitz, and H. A. Smythe. 1990. Fibromyalgia in human immunodeficiency virus infection. *Journal of Rheumatology* 17:1202-1206.

Campbell, S. M., S. Clark, E. A. Tindall, M. E. Forehand, and R. M. Bennett. 1983. Clinical characteristics of fibrositis I: A "blinded," controlled study of symptoms and tender points. *Arthritis and Rheumatism* 26(7):817-825.

Cannon, J. G., and C. A. Dinarello. 1985. Increased plasma interleukin-1 activity in women after ovulation. *Science* 227:1247-1249.

Caro, X. 1984. Immunofluorescent detection of IgG at the dermal-epidermal junction in patients with apparent fibrositis syndrome. *Arthritis and Rheumatism* 27:1174-1179.

Caro, X. 1994. ACR review part II: A metabolic hypothesis. *Fibromyalgia Network* 25(April):7. Edited by Kristin Thorson. Bakersfield, CA: Health Information Network.

Caruso, I., P. S. Puttini, M. Cazzola, V. Azzolini. 1990. Double-blind study of 5-hydroxytryptophan versus placebo in the treatment of primary fibromyalgia syndrome. *Journal of International Medical Research* 18:201-209.

Chrousos, G. P., and P. W. Gold. 1992. The concepts of stress and stress system disorders: Overview of physical and behavioral homeostasis. *Journal of the American Medical Association* 267:1244-1252.

Clark, S., S. M. Campbell, M. E. Forehand, E. A. Tindall, and R. M. Bennett. 1985. Clinical characteristics of fibrositis II: A "blinded" controlled study using standard psychological tests. *Arthritis and Rheumatism* 28:132-137.

Clark, S., E. Tindall, R. M. Bennett. 1985. A double-blind crossover trial of prednisone versus placebo in the treatment of fibrositis. *Journal of Rheumatology* 12:980-983.

Clark, S. R., C. S. Burckhardt, S. Campbell, C. O'Reilly, and R. M. Bennett. 1993. Fitness characteristics and perceived exertion in women with fibromyalgia. *Journal of Musculoskeletal Pain* 1(3/4):191-197.

Clauw, D. 1994a. Annual ACR review part I: Magnesium studies. *Fibromyalgia Network* 24(Jan.):13. Edited by Kristin Thorson. Bakersfield, CA: Health Information Network.

Clauw, D. 1994b. Team Research Update. *Fibromyalgia Network* 26(July):12. Edited by Kristin Thorson. Bakersfield, CA: Health Information Network.

Colan, B. J. 1994. Addressing trigger points with the Travell technique. *Advance for Physical Therapists* 5(28):4-5.

Cott, A., W. Parkinson, M. J. Bell, J. Adachi, M. Bedard, A. Cividino, and W. Bensen. 1992. Interrater reliability of the tender point criterion for fibromyalgia. *Journal of Rheumatology* 19:1955-1959.

Crofford, L. 1993. NIH's scientific workshop on FMS paves direction for future research: Neuro-endocrine studies. *Fibromyalgia Network* 22(July):6. Written and published by Kristin Thorson. Bakersfield, CA.

Crofford, L. J., S. R. Pillemer, K. T. Kalogeras, J. M. Cash, D. Michelson, M. A. Kling, E. M. Sternberg, P. W. Gold, G. P. Chrousos, and R. L. Wilder. 1994. Hypothalamic-pituitary-adrenal axis pertur-bations in patients with fibromyalgia. *Arthritis and Rheumatism* 37(1):1583-1592.

Cuneo, R. C., F. Salomon, C. M. Wiles, R. Hesp, and P. H. Sonksen. 1991. Growth hormone treatment in growth hormone-deficient adults II: Effects on exercise performance. *Journal of Applied Physiology* 70:695-700.

Dailey, P. A., G. D. Bishop, I. J. Russell, and E. M. Fletcher. 1990. Psychological stress and the fibrositis/fibromyalgia syndrome. *Journal of Rheumatology* 17:1380-1385.

DeVries, J. H., R. J. P. Noorda, G. A. Voetberg, and E. A. Van der Veen. 1991. Growth hormone release after the sequential use of growth hormone releasing factor and exercise. *Hormone and Metabolic Research* 23:397-398.

Dinerman, H., and A. C. Steere. 1992. Lyme disease associated with fibromyalgia. *Annals of Internal Medicine* 117:281-285.

Eisinger, J., A. Plantamurs, and T. Ayavou. 1994. Glycolysis abnormalities in fibromyalgia. *Journal of the American College of Nutrition* 13:144-148.

Elert, J. E., S. B. Rantapaa-Dahqvist, K. Henriksson-Larsen, R. Lorentson, and B. U. C. Gerdle. 1992. Muscle performance, electromyography and fibre type composition in fibromyalgia and work-related myalgia. *Scandinavian Journal of Rheumatology* 21:28-34.

Erspamer, V. 1966. Occurrence of indolealkylamines in nature. In *Handbook of Experimental Pharmacology,* edited by O. Eickerland and A. Farah, 132-181. Berlin: Springer-Verlag.

Essert, M. 1994. Water fitness: Managing your body. *Fibromyalgia Frontiers* 2(4):11-12. Edited by Tamara Liller. Centreville, VA.

Ferraccioli, G., L. Ghirelli, F. Scita, M. Nolli, M. Mozzori, S. Fontana, M. Scorsonelli, A. Tridenti, and C. DeRisio. 1987. EMG biofeedback training in fibromyalgia syndrome. *Journal of Rheumatology* 14(4):820-825.

Few, J. D. 1974. Effect of exercise on the secretion and metabolism of cortisol in man. *Journal of Endocrinology* 62:341-353.

Fischer, A. A. 1987. Pressure algometry over normal muscles: Standard values, validity and reproducibility of pressure threshold. *Pain* 30:115-126.

Frederickson, L. 1988. *Confronting mitral valve prolapse syndrome.* San Marcos, CA: Slawson Communications.

Gerster, J. C., and A. Hadj-Djilani. 1984. Hearing and vestibular abnormalities in primary fibrositis syndrome. *Journal of Rheumatology* 11(5):678-680.

Gibson, S. J., G. O. Littlejohn, M. M. Gorman, R. D. Helme, and G. Granges. 1994. Altered heat pain thresholds and cerebral event-related potentials following painful carbon dioxide laser stimulation in subjects with fibromyalgia syndrome. *Pain* 58:185-193.

Goldberg, S. 1992. *Clinical biochemistry made ridiculously simple.* Miami: Medmaster.

Goldenberg, D. L. 1986. Psychologic studies in fibrositis. *American Journal of Medicine* 81(suppl 3A):67-70.

Goldenberg, D. L. 1989. A review of the role of tricyclic medications in the treatment of fibromyalgia syndrome. *Journal of Rheumatology* 19(suppl Nov):137-9.

Goldenberg, D. L. 1994a. Fibromyalgia and chronic fatigue syndrome. *Journal of Musculoskeletal Pain* 2(3):51-55.

Goldenberg, D. L. 1994b. Medications/clinical trials in fibromyalgia. *Journal of Musculoskeletal Pain* 2(3):135-142.

Goldenberg, D. L., D. T. Felson, and H. Dinerman. 1986. A randomized, controlled trial of amitriptyline and naproxen in the treatment of patients with fibromyalgia. *Arthritis and Rheumatism* 29:1371-1377.

Goldenberg, D. L., K. H. Kaplan, M. G. Nadeau, C. Brodeur, S. Smith, and C. H. Schmid. 1994. A controlled study of a stress-reduction, cognitive-behavioral treatment program in fibromyalgia. *Journal of Musculoskeletal Pain* 2(2):53-66.

Goldenberg, D. L., R. W. Simms, A. Geiger, and A. L. Komaroff. 1989. Most patients with chronic fatigue syndrome have fibromyalgia. *Arthritis and Rheumatism* 32(4, suppl):547(abstract).

Goldstein, J. 1993a. Medical neurobiology of CFS and FMS conference review part II: Searching for answers. *Fibromyalgia Network* 23(Oct.):10. Written and published by Kristin Thorson. Bakersfield, CA: Health Information Network.

Goldstein, J. 1993b. Medical neurobiology of CFS and FMS conference review part II: Pairing up theory with data. *Fibromyalgia Network* 23(Oct.):11. Written and published by Kristin Thorson. Bakersfield, CA: Health Information Network.

Gowers, W. R. 1904. Lumbago and its analogues. *British Medical Journal* 1:117-121.

Griep, E. N., J. W. Boersma, and E. R. deKloet. 1993. Evidence for neuroendocrine disturbance following physical exercise in primary fibromyalgia syndrome. *Journal of Musculoskeletal Pain* 1(3/4):217-222.

Gronblad, M., J. Nykanen, E. Kanttinen, E. Jarvinen, and T. Helve. 1993. The effect of zopicine on sleep quality, morning stiffness, widespread tenderness and pain and general discomfort in primary fibromyalgia patients: A double blind randomized trial. *Clinical Rheumatism* 12:186-191 (abstract).

Hader, N. 1994. The immune system in FMS. *Fibromyalgia Network* 24(Jan.):11. Edited by Kristin Thorson. Bakersfield, CA: Health Information Network.

Hagberg, J. M. 1986. Central and peripheral adaptations to training in patients with coronary artery disease. *Biochemistry of Exercise* VI 16:267-277.

Hamon, M., E. Collin, D. Chantral, G. Daval, D. Verge, S. Bourgoin, and F. Cesselin. 1990. Serotonin receptors and the modulation of pain. In *Serotonin and Pain,* edited by J. M. Besson, 53-72. Excerpta Medica: Amsterdam.

Henriksson, K. 1993. Pathogenesis of fibromyalgia. *Journal of Musculoskeletal Pain* 1(3/4):3-16.

Herisson, C., L. Simon, J. Touchon, and M. Billiard. 1989. Sleeping disorders, fibrositis and mianserin treatment. *Arthritis and Rheumatism* 32 (4, suppl):570 (abstract).

Heuser, G. 1993. Medical neurobiology of CFS and FMS conference review part II. *Fibromyalgia Network* 23(Oct.):12. Written and published by Kristin Thorson. Bakersfield, CA: Health Information Network.

Hiltz, D. 1990. Clinical thermography. *Clinical Management* 10(2):28-29.

Holl, R. W., M. L. Hartman, J. D. Veldhuis, W. M. Taylor, and M. O. Thorner. 1991. Thirty-second sampling of plasma growth hormone in man: Correlation with sleep stages. *Journal of Clinical Endocrinology and Metabolism* 72:854-861.

Hong, C., Y. Chen, C. H. Pon, and J. Yu. 1993. Immediate effects of various physical medicine modalities on pain threshold of an active myofascial trigger point. *Journal of Musculoskeletal Pain* 1(2):37-54.

Hubbard, D. R., and G. M. Berkoff. 1993. Myofascial trigger points show spontaneous needle EMG activity. *Spine* 18:1803-1807.

Hudson, J. I., and H. G. Pope, Jr. 1995. Does childhood sexual abuse cause fibromyalgia? (editorial). *Arthritis and Rheumatism* 38:161-163.

Ibrahim, G. H., A. A. Essam, and F. J. Kottke. 1974. Interstitial myofibrositis: Serum and muscle enzymes and lactate dehydrogenase isoenzymes. *Archives of Physical Medicine and Rehabilitation* 55:23-28.

Isomeri, R., M. Mikkelson, P. Latikka, and K. Kammonen. 1993. Effects of amitriptyline and cardiovascular fitness training on pain in patients with primary fibromyalgia. *Journal of Musculoskeletal Pain* 1(3/4):253-260.

Jackson, M. J., D. A. Jones, and R. H. T. Edwards. 1984. Experimental skeletal muscle damage: The nature of the calcium-activated degenerative process. *European Journal of Clinical Investigation* 14:369-374.

Jacobsen, S., E. M. Bartels, and B. Danneskiold-Samsøe. 1991. Single cell morphology of muscle in patients with chronic muscle pain. *Scandinavian Journal of Rheumatology* 20:335-343.

Jacobsen, S., L. T. Jensen, M. Foldager, and B. Danneskiold-Samsøe. 1990. Primary fibromyalgia: Clinical parameters in relation to serum procollagen type III amino-terminal peptide. *British Journal of Rheumatology* 29:174-177.

Kalyan-Raman, U. P., K. Kalyan-Raman, M. B. Yunus, and A. T. Masi. 1984. Muscle pathology in primary fibromyalgia: A light microscopic, histochemical and ultrastructural study. *Journal of Rheumatology* 11(6):808-813.

Kamper-Jorgensen, F., L. A. Andreassen, D. Bruusgaard, B. Danneskiold-Samsøe, A. T. Masi, J. Morgall, and R. M. Bennett. 1992. Consensus document on fibromyalgia: The Copenhagen declaration. *Journal of Musculoskeletal Pain* 1(3/4):295-308.

Klug, G. A., E. McAuley, and S. Clark. 1989. Factors influencing the development and maintenance of aerobic fitness: Lessons applicable to the fibrositis syndrome. *Journal of Rheumatology* 16(suppl, 19):30-39.

Komaroff, A. L., D. Buchwald. 1991. Symptoms and signs of chronic fatigue syndrome. *Review of Infectious Diseases* 13:58-511.

Kotulak, R. 1994. How the brain keeps itself fit. *Chicago Tribune* September 18, Section 1:11-13.

Kravitz, H. M., R. S. Katz, N. Helmke, H. Jeffries, J. Bukovsky, and J. Fawcett. 1994. Alprazolam and ibuprofen in the treatment of fibromyalgia: Report of a double-blind placebo-controlled study. *Journal of Musculoskeletal Pain* 2(10):3-27.

Kravitz, H. M., R. Katz, E. Kot, N. Helmke, and J. Fawcett. 1992. Biochemical clues to a fibromyalgia-depression link: Imipramine binding in patients with fibromyalgia or depression and in healthy controls. *Journal of Rheumatology* 19:1428-1432.

Krueger, J. M., and L. Johannsen. 1988. *Bacterial products, cytokines and sleep, molecular mimicry in health and disease,* edited by A. Lenmark, T. Dyeberg, L. Terenius, and B. Hokfelt, 35-46. Amsterdam: Elsevier Science Publishers.

Leadbetter, W. 1992. Cell matrix response in tendon injury. *Clinics in Sports Medicine* 11(3):533-578.

Leathwood, P. D. 1987. Tryptophan availability and serotonin synthesis. *Proceedings of the Nutrition Society* 46:143-156.

Leventhal, L. J., S. J. Naides, and B. Freundlich. 1991. Fibromyalgia ... rvovirus infection. *Arthritis and Rheumatism* 34:1319-1324.

Lewis, T., G. W. Pickering, and P. Rothschild. 1931. Observations upon muscular pain in intermittent claudication. *Heart* 15:359-383.

Loveless, M. 1994. Infectious disease viewpoint. *Fibromyalgia Network* 25(Apr.):10. Edited by Kristin Thorson. Bakersfield, CA: Health Information Network.

Lue, F. A. 1994. Sleep in fibromyalgia. *Journal of Musculoskeletal Pain* 2(3):89-100.

Lund, N., A. Bengtsson, P. Thorborg. 1986. Muscle tissue oxygen pressure in primary fibromyalgia. *Scandinavian Journal of Rheumatology* 15:165-173.

Lundberg, U., and M. Frankenhaeuser. 1980. Pituitary-adrenal and sympathetic-adrenal correlates of distress and effort. *Journal of Psychosomatic Research* 24:125-130.

Mackinnon, L. T. 1989. Exercise and natural killer cells: What is the relationship? *Sports Medicine* 7:141-149.

McCain, G. A., and K. S. Tilbe. 1989. Diurnal hormone variation in fibromyalgia syndrome: A comparison with rheumatoid arthritis. *Journal of Rheumatology* (suppl, 19):154-157.

McCain, G. A., D. A. Bell, F. M. Mai, and P. D. Halliday. 1988. A controlled study of the effects of a supervised cardiovascular fitness training program on the manifestations of fibromyalgia. *Arthritis and Rheumatism* 31:1135-1141.

Melzack, R. 1981. Myofascial trigger points: Relation to acupuncture and mechanisms of pain. *Archives of Physical Medicine and Rehabilitation* 62:114-117.

Mengshoel, A. M., and Ø. Førre. 1993. Physical fitness training in patients with fibromyalgia. *Journal of Musculoskeletal Pain* 1(3/4):267-272.

Mense, S., and M. Stahnke. 1983. Contraction-sensitive fine muscle afferents. *Journal of Physiology* (London) 342:383-397.

Moldofsky, H. 1990. Sleep problems and what to do. Lecture at National Seminar on Fibrositis/Fibromyalgia, April. Columbus, Ohio.

Moldofsky, H. 1992. Sleep physiology. *Fibromyalgia Network* 18(July):5. Written and published by Kristin Thorson. Bakersfield, CA: Health Information Network.

Moldofsky, H. 1993. A chronobiologic theory of fibromyalgia. *Journal of Musculoskeletal Pain* 1(3/4):53-59.

Moldofsky, H. 1994. ACR review part II: A metabolic hypotheses. *Fibromyalgia Network* 25(Apr.):4. Edited by Kristin Thorson. Bakersfield, CA: Health Information Network.

Moldofsky, H., and F. Lue. 1980. The relationship of alpha and delta EEG frequencies to pain and mood in fibrositis patients treated with chlorpromazine and L-tryptophan. *Electroencephalography and Clinical Neurophysiology* 50:71-80.

Moldofsky, H., F. A. Lue, J. R. Davidson, and R. M. Gorczynski. 1989. Effects of sleep deprivation on human immune functions. *FASEB Journal* 3:1972-1977.

Moldofsky, H., F. A. Lue, J. Eisen, E. Keystone, and R. M. Gorczynski. 1986. The relationship of interleukin-1 and immune functions to sleep in humans. *Psychosomatic Medicine* 48:309-318.

Moldofsky, H., and P. Scarisbrick. 1976. Induction of neurasthenic musculoskeletal pain syndrome by selective sleep stage deprivation. *Psychosomatic Medicine* 38:25-44.

Moldofsky, H., P. Scarisbrick, R. England, and H. A. Smythe. 1975. Musculoskeletal symptoms and non-REM sleep disturbance in patients with "fibrositis syndrome" and healthy subjects. *Psychosomatic Medicine* 34:341-351.

Mountz, J., and L. Bradley. 1994. Annual ACR review part I: Brain scans. *Fibromyalgia Network* 24(Jan.):12. Edited by Kristin Thorson. Bakersfield, CA: Health Information Network.

Murphy, R. 1990. Exercise and athletics. Lecture at National Seminar on Fibrositis/Fibromyalgia, April. Columbus, Ohio.

Nash, P., M. Chard, and B. Hagleman. 1989. Chronic Coxsackie B infection mimicking primary fibromyalgia. *Journal of Rheumatology* 16:1506-1508.

Nørregaard, J., P. M. Bülow, and B. Danneskiold-Samsøe. 1994. Muscle strength, voluntary activation, twitch properties, and endurance in patients with fibromyalgia. *Journal of Neurology, Neurosurgery and Psychiatry* 57:1106-1111.

Nørregaard, J., P. M. Bülow, J. Mehlsen, and B. Danneskiold-Samsøe. 1994a. Biochemical changes in relation to a maximal exercise test in patients with fibromyalgia. *Clinical Physiology* 14:159-167.

Nørregaard, J., M. Harreby, K. Amris, J. Bangsbo, E. M. Bartels, and B. Danneskiold-Samsøe. 1994b. Single cell morphology and high-energy phosphate levels in quadriceps muscles from patients with fibromyalgia. *Journal of Musculoskeletal Pain* 2(2):45-52.

Pellegrino, M. W., D. Van Fossen, C. Gordon, J. M. Ryan, and G. W. Waylonis. 1989. Prevalence of mitral valve prolapse in primary fibromyalgia: A pilot investigation. *Archives of Physical Medicine and Rehabilitation* 70:541-543.

Pellegrino, M. W., G. W. Waylonis, and A. Sommer. 1989. Familial occurrence of primary fibromyalgia. *Archives of Physical Medicine and Rehabilitation* 70:61-63.

Peroutka, S. J. 1990. 5-hydroxtryptomine receptor subtypes. *Pharmacology and Toxicology* 67:373-383.

Piercey, M. F., L. A. Schroeder, K. Folkers, J. C. Xu, and J. Hong. 1981. Sensory and motor functions of spinal cord substance P. *Science* 214:1361-1362.

Quimby, L. G., G. M. Grotwick, C. D. Whitney, and S. R. Block. 1989. A randomized trial of cyclobenzaprine for the treatment of fibromyalgia. *Journal of Rheumatology* (Suppl)19:140-3.

Reichley, M. L. 1995. Aquatic, land therapy provide functional mobility for patients with fibromyalgia. *Advance for Physical Therapists* Sept. 25:8, 22.

Reilly, P. A., and G. O. Littlejohn. 1993a. Fibromyalgia: The wheel reinvented? *Journal of Musculoskeletal Pain* 1(2):5-17.

Reilly, P. A., and G. O. Littlejohn. 1993b. Diurnal variation in the symptoms and signs of the fibromyalgia syndrome (FS). *Journal of Musculoskeletal Pain* 1:(3/4):237-243.

Reynolds, M. D. 1983. The development of the concept of fibrositis. *Journal of the History of Medicine and Allied Sciences* 38:5-35.

Reynolds, W. J., H. Moldofsky, P. Saskin, and F. A. Lue. 1991. The effects of cyclobenzaprine on sleep physiology and symptoms in patients with fibromyalgia. *Journal of Rheumatology* 18:452-454.

Rodbard, S. 1975. Pain associated with muscular activity. *American Heart Journal* 90:84-92.

Romano, T. 1994. Annual ACR review part I: Brain scans. *Fibromyalgia Network* 24(Jan.):12. Edited by Kristin Thorson. Bakersfield, CA: Health Information Network.

Rubin, B. 1994. The clinical diagnosis of fibromyalgia. *Journal of Musculoskeletal Pain* 2(1):63-71.

Russell, I. J. 1992. Chronic fatigue syndrome and the brain, conference review—Research studies. *Fibromyalgia Network* 18(July):6. Written and published by Kristin Thorson. Bakersfield, CA: Health Information Network.

Russell, I. J. 1993a. A new journal. *Journal of Musculoskeletal Pain* 1(1):1-7.

Russell, I. J. 1993b. NIH's scientific workshop on FMS paves direction for future research: Metabolic studies. *Fibromyalgia Network* 22(July):5-6. Written and published by Kristin Thorson. Bakersfield, CA: Health Information Network.

Russell, I. J. 1994a. ACR review part II, a metabolic hypothesis: Brain/pituitary influences. *Fibromyalgia Network* 25(April):6. Edited by Kristin Thorson. Bakersfield, CA: Health Information Network.

Russell, I. J. 1994b. ACR review part II, a metabolic hypothesis: Substance P. *Fibromyalgia Network* 25(April):5. Edited by Kristin Thorson. Bakersfield, CA: Health Information Network.

Russell, I. J. 1994c. Current clinical status and needs assessment. Congressional Record, testimony to the U.S. House of Representatives Appropriations Subcommittee on Labor, Health and Human Services, February 1, Washington, DC.

Russell, I. J. 1994d. Pathogenesis of fibromyalgia: The neurohormonal hypothesis. *Journal of Musculoskeletal Pain* 2(1):73-86.

Russell, I. J., C. L. Bowden, J. Michalek, E. Fletcher, and G. A. Hester. 1987. Imipramine receptor density on platelets of patients with fibrositis syndrome: Correlation with disease severity and response to therapy. *Arthritis and Rheumatism* 30:S63.

Russell, I. J., E. M. Fletcher, J. E. Michalek, P. C. McBroom, and G. G. Hester. 1991. Treatment of primary fibrositis/fibromyalgia syndrome with ibuprofen and alprazolam: A double-blind, placebo-controlled study. *Arthritis and Rheumatism* 34(5):552-560.

Russell, I. J., J. E. Michalek, G. A. Vipraio, E. M. Fletcher, M. A. Javors, and C. A. Bowden. 1992a. Platelet 3H-imipramine uptake receptor density and serum serotonin levels in patients with fibromyalgia/fibrositis syndrome. *Journal of Rheumatology* 19:104-109.

Russell, I. J., J. E. Michalek, G. A. Vipraio, E. M. Fletcher, and K. Wall. 1989. Serum amino acids in fibrositis/fibromyalgia syndrome. *Journal of Rheumatology* 19:158-163.

Russell, I. J., M. D. Orr, B. Littman, G. A. Vipraio, D. Alboukrek, J. E. Michalek, Y. Lopez, and F. MacKillip. 1994. Elevated cerebrospinal fluid levels of substance P in patients with the fibromyalgia syndrome. *Arthritis and Rheumatism* 37(11):1593-1601.

Russell, I. J., H. Vaerøy, M. Javors, and F. Nyberg. 1992b. Cerebrospinal fluid biogenic amine metabolites in fibromyalgia/fibrositis syndrome and rheumatoid arthritis. *Arthritis and Rheumatism* 35: 550-556.

Russell, I. J., and G. A. Vipraio. 1993. Red cell nucleotide (RCN) abnormalities in fibromyalgia syndrome. *Arthritis and Rheumatism* 36(9):5223.

Russell, I. J., G. A. Vipraio, and I. Acworth. 1993. Abnormalities in central nervous system metabolism of tryptophan to 3-hydroxy kynurenine (OHKY) in fibromyalgia syndrome. *Arthritis and Rheumatism* 36(9):5222.

Russell, I. J., G. A. Vipraio, W. W. Morgan, and C. L. Bowden. 1986. Is there a metabolic basis for the fibrositis syndrome? *American Journal of Medicine* 81:50-56.

Russell, I. J., G. A. Vipraio, Z. Tovar, J. Michalek, and E. Fletcher. 1988. Abnormal natural killer cell activity in fibrositis syndrome is responsive in vitro to IL-2. *Arthritis and Rheumatism* 31:524 (abstract).

Schluerderberg, A., S. E. Straus, P. Peterson, S. Blumenthal, A. L. Komaroff, S. B. Spring, A. Landay, and D. Buchwald. 1992. Definition and medical outcome assessment. *Annals of Internal Medicine* 117:325-331.

Schroder, H. D., A. M. Drewes, and A. Andreasen. 1993. Muscle biopsy in fibromyalgia. *Journal of Musculoskeletal Pain* 1(3/4): 165-169.

Schuessler, G., and J. Konermann. 1993. Psychomatic aspects of primary fibromyalgia syndrome (PFS). *Journal of Musculoskeletal Pain* 1(3/4):229-236.

Schwenk, T. L. 1992. Fibromyalgia and chronic fatigue syndrome: Solving diagnostic and therapeutic dilemmas. *Modern Medicine* 60:50-57.

Scudds, R. A., G. A. McCain, G. B. Rollman, and M. Harth. 1989. Improvements in pain responsiveness in patients with fibrositis after successful treatment with amitriptyline. *Journal of Rheumatology* (Suppl 19):98-103.

Shealy, C. N. 1987. Vitamin B6 and other vitamin levels in chronic pain patients. *Clinical Journal of Pain* 2:203-204.

Sietsema, K. E., D. M. Cooper, M. R. Leibling, and J. S. Louie. 1993. Oxygen uptake during exercise in patients with primary fibromyalgia. *Journal of Rheumatology* 20:860-5.

Silverman, S. 1994. ACR review part II: A metabolic hypothesis. *Fibromyalgia Network* 25(April):6. Edited by Kristin Thorson. Bakersfield, CA: Health Information Network.

Simms, R. W. 1994. Muscle studies in fibromyalgia syndrome. *Journal of Musculoskeletal Pain* 2(3):117-123.

Simms, R. W., C. A. F. Zerbini, N. Ferrante, D. Felson, and D. E. Craven. 1992. Fibromyalgia syndrome in patients infected with human immunodeficiency virus. *American Journal of Medicine* 92:368-374.

Smythe, H. 1986. Tender points: Evaluation of concepts of the fibrositis/fibromyalgia syndrome. *American Journal of Medicine* 81(suppl 3A):2-6.

Starlanyl, D. J. 1994. Comment on the article by Hong, Chen, Pon, and Yu: Immediate effects of various physical medicine modalities on pain threshold of an active myofascial trigger point. *Journal of Musculoskeletal Pain* 2(2):141-142.

Steere, A. C., E. Taylor, G. L. McHugh, and E. L. Logigan. 1993. The overdiagnosis of Lyme disease. *Journal of the American Medical Association* 269:1812-1816.

Straus, S. E. 1994. Chronic fatigue syndrome. *Journal of Musculoskeletal Pain* 2(3):57-63.

Taylor, M. L., D. R. Trotter, and M. E. Csuka. 1995. The prevalence of sexual abuse in females with fibromyalgia syndrome. *Arthritis and Rheumatism* 38:229-234.

Travell, J., and S. H. Rinzler. 1952. The myofascial genesis of pain. *Postgraduate Medicine* 11:425-434.

Travell, J. G., and D. G. Simons. 1983. *Myofascial pain and dysfunction: The trigger point manual, vol 1*. Baltimore: Williams and Wilkins.

Travell, J. G., and D. G. Simons. 1992. *Myofascial pain and dysfunction: Trigger point manual, vol. 2*. Baltimore: Williams and Wilkins.

Tunks, E., J. Crook, G. Norman, and S. Kalaker. 1988. Tender points in fibromyalgia. *Pain* 34:11-19.

Vaerøy, H., R. Helle, Ø. Førre, E. Kåss, and L. Terenius. 1988. Elevated CSF levels of substance P and high incidence of Raynaud phenomenon in patients with fibromyalgia: New features for diagnosis. *Pain* 32:21-26.

Vaerøy, H., Z. G. Qiao, L. Mørkrid, and Ø. Førre. 1989. Altered sympathetic nervous system response in patients with fibromyalgia (fibrositis syndrome). *Journal of Rheumatology* 16(11):1460-1465.

van Denderen, J. C., J. W. Boersma, P. Zeinstra, A. P. Hollander, and B. R. van Neerbos. 1992. Physiological effects of exhaustive physical exercise in primary fibromyalgia syndrome (PFS): Is PFS a disorder of neuroendocrine reactivity? *Scandinavian Journal of Rheumatology* 21:35-7.

Verstapen, F. T. J., H. M. S. Van Santen-Hoeufft, S. van Sloun, P. H. Bolwijn, S. Vander Linden. 1995. Fitness characteristics of female patients with fibromyalgia. *Journal of Musculoskeletal Pain* 3(3):45-58.

Wagenmakers, A. J. M., J. H. Coakley, and R. H. T. Edwards. 1988. The metabolic consequences of reduced habitual activities in patients with muscle pain and disease. *Ergonomics* 31(1):1519-1527.

Waylonis, G. W. 1990. Exercise therapy in fibromyalgia. Lecture at National Seminar Fibrositis/Fibromyalgia, April. Columbus, Ohio.

Waylonis, G. W., P. G. Ronan, and C. Gordon. 1994. A profile of fibromyalgia in occupational environments. *American Journal of Physical Medicine and Rehabilitation* 73(2):112-115.

Weltman, A., J. Y. Weltman, R. Schurrer, W. S. Evans, J. D. Veldhuis, and A. D. Rogol. 1992. Endurance training amplifies the pulsatile release of growth hormone: Effects of training intensity. *Journal of Applied Physiology* 72:2188-2196.

Whelton, C. L., I. Salit, and H. Moldofsky. 1992. Sleep, Epstein-Barr virus infection, musculoskeletal pain, and depressive symptoms in chronic fatigue syndrome. *Journal of Rheumatology* 19:939-943.

White, D. M., and R. D. Helme. 1985. Release of substance P from peripheral nerve terminals following electrical stimulation of the sciatic nerve. *Brain Research* 336:27-31.

White, K. P., G. A. McCain, and E. Tunks. 1993. The effects of changing the painful stimulus upon dolorimetry scores in patients with fibromyalgia. *Journal of Musculoskeletal Pain* 1(1):43-58.

Wolfe, F. 1993a. Disability and the dimensions of distress in fibromyalgia. *Journal of Musculoskeletal Pain* 1(2):65-87.

Wolfe, F. 1993b. Fibromyalgia: On diagnosis and certainty. *Journal of Musculoskeletal Pain* 1(3/4):17-35.

Wolfe, F. 1994. Aspects of the epidemiology of fibromyalgia. *Journal of Musculoskeletal Pain* 2(3):65-77.

Wolfe, F., K. Ross, J. Anderson, I. J. Russell, and L. Hebert. 1995. The prevalence and characteristics of fibromyalgia in the general population. *Arthritis and Rheumatism* 38:19-28.

Wolfe, F., H. A. Smythe, M. B. Yunus, R. M. Bennett, C. Bombardier, D. L. Goldenberg, P. Tugwell, S. M. Campbell, M. Abeles, P. Clark, A. G. Fam, S. J. Farber, J. J. Fiechtner, C. M. Franklin, R. A. Gatter, D. Hamaty, J. Lessard, A. S. Lichtbroun, A. T. Masi, G. A. McCain, W. J. Reynolds, T. J. Tomano, I. J. Russell, and R. P. Sheon. 1990. The American College of Rheumatology 1990 criteria for the classification of fibromyalgia. Report of the Multicenter Criteria Committee. *Arthritis and Rheumatism* 33(2):160-172.

Yunus, M. B. 1993. NIH's scientific workshop on FMS paves direction for future research: Neuro-endocrine studies. *Fibromyalgia Network* 22(July):6. Written and published by Kristin Thorson. Bakersfield, CA: Health Information Network.

Yunus, M. B. 1994. Psychological factors in fibromyalgia syndrome: An overview. *Journal of Musculoskeletal Pain* 2(1):87-91.

Yunus, M. B., T. A. Ahles, T. C. Aldag, and A. T. Masi. 1991. Relationship of clinical features with psychological status in primary fibromyalgia. *Arthritis and Rheumatism* 34:15-21.

Yunus, M. B., J. W. Dailey, J. C. Aldag, A. T. Masi, and P. C. Jobe. 1992. Plasma tryptophan and other amino acids in primary fibromyalgia: A controlled study. *Journal of Rheumatology* 19:90-94.

Yunus, M. B., A. T. Masi, and J. C. Aldag. 1989. Short-term effects of ibuprofen in primary fibromyalgia syndrome: A double-blind, placebo controlled trial. *Journal of Rheumatology* 16:527-532.

Yunus, M. B., A. T. Masi, J. J. Calabro, K. A. Miller, and S. L. Feigenbaum. 1981. Primary fibromyalgia (fibrositis): Clinical study of 50 patients with matched normal controls. *Seminars in Arthritis and Rheumatism* 11:151-171.

Zacharkow, D. 1994. Sitting posture: The overlooked factor in carpal tunnel syndrome. *Advance for Physical Therapists* May 16:8-9, 17.

Zidar, J., E. Bäckman, A. Bengtsson, and K. G. Henriksson. 1990. Quantitative EMG and muscle tension in painful muscles in fibromyalgia. *Pain* 40(3):249-254.